Praise

Casey Hough's *Known for Love* is a wonderful one-volume resource that Christians need in this urgent hour. With the heart of a pastor and the mind of a professor, Casey brings great interpretive care to arrive at conclusions that are as full of grace as they are of truth.

ANDREW T. WALKER
Associate Professor of Christian Ethics and Public Theology, The Southern Baptist Theological Seminary

Known for Love by Casey Hough is an essential guide for any disciple of Jesus seeking to navigate the intersection of faith and LGBTQ relationships with grace and integrity. With compassion and biblical wisdom, Hough invites readers to embrace a posture of grace and love that rejoices in truth. This book offers a timely and much-needed perspective, equipping readers to be winsome ambassadors for Christ. It is a must-read for anyone seeking to love God and others well as they seek to live as disciples of Jesus.

EVAN POSEY
Executive Vice President and Provost Luther Rice College and Seminary

Engaging LGBT friends and family with both truth and grace is one of the most important issues of our age. Casey Hough outlines a thorough and biblical case for the historic Christian sexual ethic while also giving wise and pastoral guidelines for living this out faithfully in our age. This is a resource every Christian should have, and every church should have in bulk.

DANIEL DARLING
Director of the Land Center for Cultural Engagement and author of several books, including *The Dignity Revolution, Agents of Grace*, and *A Way with Words*

Anthropology is the issue of our lifetime. People endlessly debate over views of gender and sexuality. And it's not going to stop. As a pastor, I'm always looking for trustworthy and helpful resources to put into the hands of other leaders and church members. As a father, I'm always wanting to help my children work through the real issues they'll face living as Christians in a world with wildly different values and beliefs than theirs. *Known for Love* does both. Casey Hough helps Christians live by Jesus' call to love our neighbors without compromising biblical truth.

ERIK REED
Lead Pastor of The Journey Church in Lebanon, TN; founder of Knowing Jesus Ministries

There is a false dichotomy in our cultural moment that claims either you bless and affirm someone's same-sex desires, or you are a homophobic bigot. Sadly, the result is that many evangelicals have chosen to remain silent on the matter altogether in order to resist labels and pressures they are unwilling to handle. The church needs more resources to equip believers in how they can avoid the false dichotomy. We must be clear on God's design, and also unwavering in love of neighbor. Those postures are not at odds with one another, and Casey Hough has helped us to how to be biblical in what I believe is the greatest matter of confusion in our culture today.

DEAN INSERRA
Lead Pastor, City Church, Tallahassee; author of *The Unsaved Christian*

KNOWN

FOR

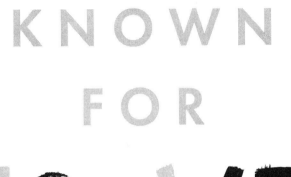

Loving Your LGBTQ Family & Friends

Without Compromising Biblical Truth

CASEY B. HOUGH

MOODY PUBLISHERS
CHICAGO

All Scripture quotations, unless otherwise noted, are taken from the Holy Bible, New International Version®, NIV®. Copyright ©1973, 1978, 1984, 2011 by Biblica, Inc.™ Used by permission of Zondervan. All rights reserved worldwide. www.zondervan.com The "NIV" and "New International Version" are trademarks registered in the United States Patent and Trademark Office by Biblica, Inc.™

Scripture quotations marked (ESV) are from the ESV® Bible (The Holy Bible, English Standard Version®), © 2001 by Crossway, a publishing ministry of Good News Publishers. Used by permission. All rights reserved. The ESV text may not be quoted in any publication made available to the public by a Creative Commons license. The ESV may not be translated in whole or in part into any other language.

Emphasis to Scripture has been added.

Edited by Pamela J. Pugh
Interior design: Brandi Davis
Cover design: Thinkpen Design
Cover illustration of fingerprint heart copyright © 2023 by Denis Bunin/Shutterstock (564177583). All rights reserved.
Author photo: CMadlee Photography

Library of Congress Cataloging-in-Publication Data

Names: Hough, Casey B., author.
Title: Known for love : loving your LGBTQ friends and family without compromising biblical truth / by Casey B. Hough.
Description: Chicago, IL : Moody Publishers, 2024. | Includes bibliographical references. | Summary: "In Known for Love, pastor Casey Hough provides a biblical and theological framework for thinking through the hard situations we encounter with family and friends. Drawing from a well of faithful biblical scholars, Hough provides insights for everyday Christians living in a sexually broken world. Known for Love gives us the wisdom and courage we need to live into these days with faithful and truly loving hearts"-- Provided by publisher.
Identifiers: LCCN 2023057512 (print) | LCCN 2023057513 (ebook) | ISBN 9780802433756 (paperback) | ISBN 9780802471062 (ebook)
Subjects: LCSH: Homosexuality--Religious aspects--Christianity. | Homosexuality--Biblical teaching. | Love--Religious aspects--Christianity. | Christian gay people. | Christian ethics. | BISAC: RELIGION / Christian Theology / Ethics | HEALTH & FITNESS / Sexuality
Classification: LCC BR115.H6 H75 2024 (print) | LCC BR115.H6 (ebook) | DDC 261.8/35766--dc23/eng/20240209
LC record available at https://lccn.loc.gov/2023057512
LC ebook record available at https://lccn.loc.gov/2023057513

Originally delivered by fleets of horse-drawn wagons, the affordable paperbacks from D. L. Moody's publishing house resourced the church and served everyday people. Now, after more than 125 years of publishing and ministry, Moody Publishers' mission remains the same—even if our delivery systems have changed a bit. For more information on other books (and resources) created from a biblical perspective, go to www.moodypublishers.com or write to:

Moody Publishers
820 N. LaSalle Boulevard
Chicago, IL 60610

1 3 5 7 9 10 8 6 4 2

Printed in the United States of America

This book is dedicated to my mother, Julia Kay Hough. Possibly more than anyone that I have ever known, she embodies a love for others that refuses to compromise the truth of God's Word. It is her uncompromising commitment to God's Word that shapes her love for others. Thank you for setting such a wonderful example for me, Mom.

Contents

The Aim of This Book

I write this book as a parent, a pastor, and a professor.

When I think about the challenges that my children, my congregants, and my students face, I am often overwhelmed. You might wonder, "Why focus on sex? Aren't there other circumstances that Christians face?" Yes. There are definitely other circumstances that Christians face in our present world. Yet the most common questions that I am faced with are related to living faithfully as a disciple of Christ known for love in a world that is openly hostile to the Christian faith's vision of sexuality. If I were constantly being asked questions about how to live faithfully in a world that glorifies theft, I would probably be writing this book on that topic. But my children, congregants, and students do not yet seem to be living in a world that, by and large, says that it is okay to steal from others.

Instead, I am fielding questions from grieving Christian parents whose children have bought into the lie that their bodies do not matter and that they can sleep with whomever they want to sleep with without any consequence.

I'm counseling parents whose children are confused about basic questions like, "What does it mean to be a man or a woman?"

I'm helping leaders of churches work through how to have biblical convictions about sexuality while also demonstrating the love of Christ.

I'm contributing to resources that help political leaders think through matters like freedom of speech and religious liberty that are endangered by the current trajectory of the sexual revolution.

I'm comforting grandparents whose grandchildren are abandoning the faith they once professed in favor of the faith of the sexual revolution. This is just the world that we live in right now. It is an issue that everyone is wrestling with, so if I'm going to be helpful, I must provide help where it is needed most.

This book aims to equip you to be known for love in a world that is "no friend of grace."

We do not need the world to be on our side to be faithful Christians. But we will never be faithful Christians known for love without God's grace in Christ through the Holy Spirit.

Throughout the book, we'll grapple with a graceful and loving response to the practical issues of our day in the area of sexuality. You'll see interspersed five chapters laying out a biblical-theological framework so we can have a foundation for our response. This framework will examine Creation, Crisis, Christ, Creation Regained, and, finally, Our Place in God's Redemptive Plan. Together, these topics cover the whole storyline of the Bible, and I encourage you not to miss those chapters! This framework will help us navigate some of the tougher questions about how we are called to live as believers in the New Testament. My interest is not so much in providing some "ethical answer key" for Christians. Instead, I want to equip you with a biblical foundation from which we can develop principles of engagement for a faithful Christian life of love.

It is vital for Christians to learn how to work through these matters in a principled way as the questions change from one generation to the next.

We still have a mandate from Jesus to make disciples of all nations and teach them to obey all that Christ has commanded us (Matt. 28:18–20). We still have an obligation to love the Lord our God with all our heart, soul, mind, and strength while loving our neighbors as ourselves (Matt. 22:37–40). This includes loving our neighbors who believe that our convictions about the life, death, burial, resurrection, and ascension of Jesus are ridiculous. This includes our neighbors who believe Christian sexual ethics are antiquated and oppressive. And this includes our neighbors who identify as lesbian, gay, bisexual, transgender, queer, intersex, nonbinary, or asexual.

The practical chapters woven among the framework chapters are intended to give concrete examples of how we might understand, obey, and apply God's Word in our present world. I believe such an approach is more valuable than other approaches that simply answer questions about moral issues that we are currently facing because of the speed at which our world is moving. While answers to such questions are important (and there will certainly be some found in the pages that follow), I believe that it is vital for Christians to learn how to work through these matters in a principled way as the questions change from one generation to the next.

My goal is not to pick on people who believe differently from me

11

but rather to help believers love God and others well as they seek to live as disciples of Jesus. My prayer is that it will help you follow Jesus faithfully as you love the wayward ones in your family, in your church, and in your community with the hope that you will one day be able to read the words of 1 Corinthians 6:11 and say, "And that is what some of you *were*. But you were washed, you were sanctified, you were justified in the name of the Lord Jesus Christ and by the Spirit of our God."

I write this book with full confidence in the power of the gospel of God's grace in Jesus Christ to transform lives. As you read, I ask that you do your best not to allow sentiment or public opinion to define what is true and loving. I ask that you open God's Word and taste and see for yourself. Read it with an awareness that the words on the page are the very words of God Himself. Study and handle God's Word as a servant under His Word who will interpret and apply it in a manner that will not be put to shame on the day of Jesus' return. Read it as someone who desires to be known for a love that rejoices in the truth.

CHAPTER ONE

Exploring the Biblical-Theological Framework One

CREATION: "And It Was Very Good"

A few years ago, I got into studying my family history. There was a free trial available through one of those ancestry websites, so I signed up and started digging.

During that time, I made several phone calls to my mom and dad to get details about our family. Honestly, I became a little obsessed. I toyed with the idea of sending in a DNA sample to learn more, but something about sending a swab of my spit to a stranger who would enter my information into a global database felt a little too intrusive. Anyway, I dug as deeply as I could before my trial ran out, but I eventually hit a wall. Still, I made it back to the eleventh century. Maybe one day, I will have more time and money to keep going.

As I studied my family's history, I learned things that brought me a lot of joy and others that brought me sorrow. One of the joy-filling things was seeing pictures of old properties that my ancestors likely lived on several centuries ago. In fact, I could pull up a castle that was supposedly owned by some of my ancestors. For a brief time, my kids were convinced that we still had some claim of ownership to that castle. To their disappointment, I explained that it doesn't work that way.

One of the things that brought me dismay, though, was that I had at least one relative who served as a chaplain with the Confederate Army during the Civil War. As a father of two beautiful African American daughters, it pains me to know that some of my ancestors would have viewed my children as property. I cannot change my family's history, but by God's grace, my family's future doesn't have to conform to the sins of previous generations. I'm so grateful for the transforming power of God's grace in Christ.

My study of my family's history was motivated by a desire to know more about my identity. The question that led me to sign up for that trial and spend all those hours searching through the database was, "Who am I?" There was something about knowing who I am that I believed was intimately related to how I lived in this world. Deep down, I think I was hoping to discover that I was the descendant of a long line of gospel ministers who gave their lives in service to Christ. Or maybe learn that I was related to missionaries who took the gospel to the nations. But none of that came to fruition. Instead, I learned that my family history, while special to me, is not unlike many other family histories: full of excitement and disappointment. After all, all our family histories are family histories of sinners.

Part of the problem with my study, though, is that it simply needed to go back further. If I wanted to know who I am and how I am to live in this world, then I would have to get back to the beginning of it all. I had to get back to where it all started.

IN THE BEGINNING: IMAGE BEARERS

So, what did Jesus say, believe, and teach about the beginning of humanity? In Matthew 19, when the Pharisees questioned Him about divorce, Jesus referred back to creation. The Pharisees asked, "Is it lawful for a man to divorce his wife for any and every reason?" Jesus responded, "Haven't you read that at the beginning the Creator 'made them male and female' . . . ?"

His response reveals that He understood the Creator's work as a divine revelation about God's purpose for human sexuality, gender, and marriage. Jesus continued, stating, "For this reason a man will leave his father and mother and be united to his wife, and the two will become one flesh. So they are no longer two, but one flesh . . . Therefore what God has joined together, let no one separate" (vv. 4–5).

We don't have to wonder what Jesus thought or believed about the beginning of humanity. He reveals His beliefs in this conversation. Notice how Jesus quotes approvingly from Genesis 1 and 2 as a revelation of God's purpose for humans from the beginning. We should understand these opening chapters of the Bible to reveal a Creator God who not only brings the world into existence but also orders that world for a purpose. While understanding the origins of our world as important, it is also important to take note of the order of our world from the beginning.

Old Testament scholar Sandra Richter describes this opening scene in Genesis as "God's blueprint for creation."[1] Richter explains that God can be seen creating and ordering a world of "interdependence," where both habitats and inhabitants exist according to His plan. In ancient times, both God's creation and His ordering of the world were understood to be closely related. Each aspect of creation has a role to play in the grand story that God is telling us about His purpose.

The world was not to be an empty, chaotic, formless void. God, in creating and ordering the world, reveals what He intends for His creation.

For most people of the ancient Near East, the story of God saying, "Let there be light" on the first day of creation would have pointed them not to "the creation of what physicists call light" but instead to "the setting up of the cycle of day and night—the creation of the basis for time."[2] The same thing could be said for subsequent days where the basis for weather and vegetation were established. God's creation was ordered for a purpose. Even the sequencing of the days of creation points to the importance of recognizing order and purpose in creation. The world was not to be an empty, chaotic, formless void. God, in creating and ordering the world, reveals what He intends for His creation.

In the first three days, God created and ordered the "habitats" or "kingdoms" of day and night, the sea and sky, and the dry land. Then, over the next three days, God created inhabitants that would be placed in their respective habitats. The sun and moon would "rule the day and night, the fish and birds would occupy the sea and sky, and the other creatures would inhabit the dry land."[3] The creation story, however, does not end at the beginning of the sixth day.

According to Genesis 1:26, God said, "Let us make mankind in our image, in our likeness, so that they may rule over the fish in the sea and the birds in the sky, over the livestock and all the wild animals, and over all the creatures that move along the ground." While some translations refer to "man" being created in the image of God, the language in Genesis 1:26 is intentionally collective, which means that it refers to both male and female being created in the image of God (*imago Dei*) and bearing the responsibility to rule over the rest of creation.[4] Male and female are both created in God's image, having equal dignity and playing important roles in God's plan.

Humanity, as the bearers of God's image, would enjoy a special role in creation. As John Walton, a noted scholar of the ancient Near East, wrote, "When God creates people in his image it indicates, perhaps among other things, that we are to function as his stewards over creation."[5]

Christians have debated what exactly it means to be God's image bearers, but they have not doubted the fact that humans possess a special relationship to God. Humanity enjoys a special relationship with God that no other created thing enjoys. Don't rush by the significance of being created in God's image. As one theologian put it,

> Whatever else the *imago Dei* might mean, there can be little doubt that it stands as paradigmatic of all creation in its calling to reflect or mirror God. It is an exhilarating and exalting description, intended to signify the privilege of imaging God. It is also a humbling description, reminding humankind that it is not divine, but merely an image of the Creator.[6]

What a thought, right? Humanity is unique in its relationship to God. While I love my pets, they don't bear God's image like my children. There is something very special about our relationship to God as our Creator.

With this special relationship comes certain responsibilities or tasks defined by God Himself. Humans are tasked with a special role in creation to glorify God. Think of how children will, for better or worse, reflect certain characteristics of their family. We tend to reflect what we see. And similarly, each of us, having been stamped as God's image bearers, will, even at times unknowingly, reflect aspects of His creative character in our words and deeds.

Sadly, however, our ability to perceive and reflect God's image has been significantly impacted by sin. Our vision of who God is and what He has called us to do does not come as naturally to us as it did for the first humans. This is why it is so crucial for us to return to and reflect on the beginning because who we are and how we are to live in the world is defined by our unique relationship with God Himself.

LORD AND RULER OVER ALL

If we stop reading at the end of Genesis 1, though, we will miss out on a crucial aspect of the creation story on the seventh day. According to Genesis 2:1–3, after completing His creative work, God "rested from all his work," then "blessed the seventh day and made it holy." By concluding the creation account with God's own rest from and reflection on creation, God is presented as the ultimate Lord and Ruler over creation, a theme found throughout Scripture. As the Lord over creation, God gives us our identity and tells us how we are to live to glorify Him.

In Genesis 2, we find a more detailed account of the creation of humanity with the benefit of learning more about their relationship to God and one another. Regarding humanity's relationship with God, they were free to enjoy and steward God's creation in the garden of Eden as His image bearers on earth. The only stipulation that they were given was to "not eat from the tree of the knowledge of good and evil" (Gen. 2:17). Again, I found Sandra Richter's thought on this point helpful. Commenting on the "stipulations," Richter wrote, "The blessings are many, the stipulations few. In fact, the only negative stipulation of this covenant is 'you shall not eat of the tree of the knowledge of good and evil.' On the surface this seems like a simple, even silly rule. But in reality this one edict encompasses the singular law of Eden—God is God and we are not."[7]

> Creation is the initial act and foundation of all divine revelation and therefore the foundation of all religious and ethical life as well.[8] — Herman Bavinck

We must not miss this crucial aspect of creation. While there are many debates within Christianity about the particulars of creation that will likely continue (e.g., the age of the earth, the mechanism of creation, the length of days), such debates should not prevent us from affirming certain truths about creation and their implications for our lives.[9] I fear that while such debates can be important, they can also be overly complicated, leading us to ignore the significance of creation for everyday discipleship.[10] If creation teaches us anything, it teaches us that God is unique and distinct from humanity.

As the Creator, He is Lord over His creation.

The Creator-creature distinction must be acknowledged. Without this distinction, we will not know or love God as we have been called to know and love Him, nor will we live in the world as we have been called to live. If we get the significance of the beginning wrong, we will get everything else wrong too. Jesus knew this was the case, so He pointed the Pharisees back to the beginning to answer their questions about marriage and divorce, which has profound implications for our questions about sexuality in this broken world.

AND IT WAS VERY GOOD

The implications of Genesis 1–2 for our understanding of God's world and God's Word are hard to overstate. For one, we see the goodness of creation as God intended, which ought to stir us to be good stewards of it. Those who take God's Word seriously ought to be mindful of things like animal welfare and creation care. Furthermore, Genesis 1–2 should help us see that creation is not without purpose. What God has created and ordered is not endlessly malleable. We are called to be stewards of creation, not anarchists. We are free but within boundaries. And when we violate the boundaries God has established for us within His creation, things go horribly wrong.

As we watch Jesus speak with the Pharisees, we see that things like divorce are concessions within a world that has gone bad. God's purpose in creating male and female and joining them together as one flesh in marriage is the ideal. As we have already seen, as the Lord over creation, God does more than create; He also orders His creation. And as Genesis 1:31 shows us, God's created order, before sin's entrance into the world, was "very good."

This "very good" order, as the ideal of creation, does not get erased when humanity rebels against God. Instead, it remains the divine pattern for humanity, as Jesus' interaction with the Pharisees demonstrates. While a concession in certain circumstances was made for divorce later through Moses, that does not mean that it was God's plan for His creation from the beginning. Thus, Jesus points the Pharisees back to the very good creation to teach us whom God made us to be in this world: image bearers who bring Him glory.

"GOODNESS LOOKS LIKE GOD"

Jesus' appeal to "the beginning" is a paradigm for discerning the essential goodness of our thoughts and behaviors. Among a host of other reasons, we can trust Jesus' teaching on goodness because He has definitively declared that "goodness" is found in God alone.[11]

In Luke 18:18, a certain rich man asked Jesus, "Good teacher, what must I do to inherit life?" Jesus responded, "No one is good—except God alone." Jesus did not deny His goodness as God incarnate with His response to the young man, but instead, He was correcting the misunderstanding that "goodness" can be defined by a "teacher." If we would recognize the good, then we must recognize it in relationship to God. Or, as Iain Provan puts it, "Goodness looks like God."[12]

God is the one who first utters the declaration, "and it was good." To do so, He must not only know what goodness is but also be the source of the definition of goodness. Before creation, the existence of goodness dwelt securely within the life of the triune God. In other words, when God created the world and declared it to be "good," the goodness of creation was relative to the goodness of God Himself. We can only know that something is good because of its relationship to the One who alone is good in Himself. Only God can define "good" because being "good" is part of His essence.

Much as how holiness, love, justice, righteousness, and life depend upon God for their definition, "good" finds its source in God alone. If we could appeal to someone or something outside of God to define these fundamental aspects of God's nature and creation, then the thing we appeal to would functionally have more authority than God Himself. And to appeal to a higher authority than God Himself would be to make God no god at all. Hence, Christians must heed Jesus' teaching to the rich young man and look to God alone for our understanding of the "good," especially as it relates to creation.

With each day of creation, God declared the existence and purpose of creation to be good, climaxing with Genesis 1:31, where He says, "and it was very good." These words "emphasize the perfection of the final work" of creation.[13] It is a comprehensive statement about the whole creation. Nothing that God has made is exempted from His declaration that "it was very good."

GENERAL AND SPECIAL REVELATION

When God makes such a declaration about His creation, we must recognize that such goodness is inextricably related to God's order and intention for His creation. It is not enough to acknowledge that God has created all things. God's statement presupposes that His creation conforms to His intention for creation. Another way to state this would be to say that in order for something to be good, it must conform to God's will. We can know God's will because He has graciously chosen to reveal it. But how has He revealed it? Christians have typically spoken of God's revelation of His will in two forms: general revelation (sometimes referred to as "natural revelation") and special revelation.

General revelation refers to how God has revealed Himself in creation. Theologian Michael Bird offers this definition for general (or natural) revelation: it is "the disclosure of God's existence and attributes as discerned through human intuition and as inferred from nature."[14] Even though sin has distorted our perspective of this general revelation, humans are still held accountable to God. The apostle Paul makes this point in Romans 1:20–22, where he mentions the revelation of God's invisible attributes in the things that were made.

Jesus regularly pointed to natural occurrences to make a point about who God is and how we are to live. Just think of Jesus telling the crowds to consider the lilies or watch the birds and reflect upon how God cares for them. What was the lesson to be learned? If God takes cares of flowers and birds, then you don't have anything to worry about. God's going to take care of you too. This is an example of general revelation being used by Jesus to teach us about God and about ourselves. Yet, this general revelation, while sufficient up to a point, is not sufficient for navigating this world. We need God's special revelation to know who we are and how we are to faithfully live as image bearers.

What, then, is special revelation? Again, I find theologian Michael Bird's definition helpful. Special revelation is "God's unique and supernatural communication of himself."[15] So, unlike what can be known about God through creation and human intuition, special revelation occurred through events "like the exodus or the resurrection of Christ." Furthermore, as Bird continues, it was observed through the "inspired proclamation of the prophets and apostles." Then, as most of us likely know it, special revelation occurs in the form of Scripture, which Christians understand to be "breathed-out" or "inspired" by God Himself "through human authors to produce written texts."[16]

God's special revelation is what sinful humanity needs to properly understand God, His salvation, and His intention in the world. While general revelation might point us vaguely to some of these realities, ultimately, we need God's supernatural intervention to give us wisdom. This is the same kind of revelation that the humans in the garden of Eden received as God commanded them to "be fruitful and multiply on the earth." It was God's special revelation, His very words to Adam and Eve, that revealed His will for their lives. They knew who they were and how they were to live because God had told them. And God had already declared that His creation and will for humanity were good. Very good.

RECOGNIZING THE GOOD

So, in recognizing the good, we must ask, "What is God's will? What has He revealed to us about the good?" At this point, I want it to be clear that I am using the language of "recognizing the good" instead of saying "defining the good." As the Creator God, He has already "defined the good" for us. Our task as image bearers is not to define or redefine what is good, but rather to recognize the good as He has revealed it and conform our lives to that very good design.

As we observe God's creation in Genesis 1–2, we can perceive that God ordered His creation toward life. As humanity worked the land, they would cultivate food that would sustain them in their work to expand the garden. As they enjoyed marital union, they would fulfill the mandate to "be fruitful and multiply," resulting in offspring who would carry on the image-bearing work. And they would engage in this work until the day when the whole earth was a garden filled with the presence of the Lord among His people. And this life would be good because it was the life that the good God had called His people to in His good creation. All of creation would reflect the goodness of God. But, as we will see, humanity did not trust God's definition of the good. Instead, they sought to define their own good, which ended very badly. But, as Jesus taught, we can know "the good" if we return to God, the source of all good.

Thus far, we have considered Jesus' insistence on defining the good in relation to God and viewing God's intention in creation as the paradigm by which we should assess our thoughts and actions. So, what would it look like to make such an assessment in light of these truths about creation?

We need to bring our thoughts and actions into submission to God's will as He has revealed it in creation. Doing so helps us evaluate the thoughts and actions that are prevalent within our society. For instance, when assessing whether a public policy regarding the environment or marriage is good, we should ask questions like, "How would this policy promote the flourishing of creation as God intended?" or "How does this policy promote the stability and sanctity of marriage between one man and one woman for life as God intended?"

As Christians, while we acknowledge that sin has corrupted the whole world, we also recognize that such corruption has not erased the ideals embedded within creation. As Jesus' example with the Pharisees reveals, while concessions in a fallen world might be made at certain points and even be part of our traditions, God's ideal for humanity remains. And it is very good.

———

In the next chapter, we'll continue with our theological framework to understand what has gone wrong with God's very good creation. We're going to see what this all has to do with sexuality.

CHAPTER TWO

Exploring the Biblical-Theological Framework Two

CRISIS:
Not the Way It's
Supposed to Be

D ad, I prayed that Papaw would get better, but he didn't. Why would God let him die?"

These were the words from my youngest son just hours after my father passed away. If I'm honest, I was still trying to make sense of it all too. Why does death have to be a part of this life?

My father lived a full life. He lived almost eighty-one years, enjoyed sixty-one years of marriage, and had three sons and fourteen grandchildren. And he worked right up until the weekend before he started to get sick. I spoke with him on Father's Day. I had just arrived and settled in Uganda after spending a week in South Sudan training pastors when I received the message that Dad was not feeling well and was headed to the hospital. He had a terrible headache, and his blood pressure was high. I arranged to travel back to the US that night. After a battery of tests, they determined that my dad had a bleeding stroke. As the day progressed, he became less responsive. I returned to be with my family, but within a week, he passed away surrounded by his loved ones in a crowded ICU room.

A friend that I had spoken with earlier in the week tried to prepare me for how I would feel if he didn't make it. He told me not to be surprised if I felt like a child all over again. When Dad passed away, I felt disoriented. I never realized how much stability I subconsciously drew from my father's presence. Even as an adult with five children of my own, I took my dad's availability for granted. He encouraged me through bouts of depression and discouragement in ministry. He helped me repair small engines and told me when to spread fertilizer in my yard. He taught me to hunt, fish, and drive. He instilled in me a love for good country music artists like Hank Williams Sr., George Jones, and Vince Gill. And in his own simple way, he reminded me to trust God when things were hard. But now Dad was gone. No more birthday calls. No more handshakes with his rugged, work-worn hands. No more questions about how the boys had done in the ball games. No more "Love ya, buddy" and "Be careful" signoffs from our conversations. Death had stolen these blessings from me.

I was, as my mother would say, a "mid-life blessing," which means that I was unexpected but welcomed nonetheless. I enjoyed thirty-eight years with my dad. Given how many of my friends lost their fathers early in life, I'm grateful that I had him as long as I did. Yet, losing him still hurt. People will say, "Death is just part of life," but it wasn't always this way. In terms of God's ideal for humanity, this is not how it's supposed to be.[1]

WHAT WENT WRONG?

If you believe that human life has a purpose and is not simply "the outcome of accidental collocations of atoms," then you likely perceive that something is wrong in the world.[2] Most people have categories of right and wrong, good and evil, wholeness and brokenness. One can hardly look at the world and think, "This is perfect." So, what went wrong in this world that God described as "very good"?

When we return to the beginning of Genesis, where we originally encountered God's declaration about the goodness of the created world, we find that the story continues after the creation of humanity. God created and placed humanity in the garden of Eden to expand its borders so that the relational presence of God might one day fill the whole earth.[3] Adam and Eve were to "be fruitful and multiply" while taking dominion over the earth. The only stipulation that they were given was to "not eat of the tree of the knowledge of good and evil." Simple enough, right?

While Adam and Eve could enjoy everything else that God provided them, they were told not to eat the fruit of this one particular tree. Yet, Adam and Eve did not obey.

At this point, you might be thinking, *I know all this. What does all this have to do with sexuality?* Stick with me. I promise it's important.

Instead of trusting God and His will for their lives, they listened to that ancient liar, the serpent, who told them that "they would not surely die" if they disobeyed God. Instead, they would be "like God." The serpent promised that their rebellion would lead to humanity's progress in the world. No need to listen to or obey God. But, as we continue to read, we learn that they were deceived. The progress did not come as they had hoped. As Herman Bavinck put it, "Genesis 3 does not tell the story of a 'giant step of progress' but of a human fall."[4]

By disobeying God and eating the forbidden fruit, humanity, in a sense, got what it wanted: freedom from God's order. They were deceived into believing that freedom from God would lead to true happiness, but instead, it led to great devastation and death in the world. Humanity's disobedience led to a form of liberation that brought bondage. And ever since that day, the world has been plagued by sin which leads to devastation and death. But what exactly is sin?

THE NATURE OF SIN

Theologian Thomas McCall defines sin as "whatever is opposed to God's will, as that will reflects God's holy character and as that will is expressed by God's commands."[5] He continues, stating, "Sin is fundamentally opposed to nature and reason, and it is ultimately opposed to God. The results of sin are truly catastrophic—sin wreaks havoc on our relationships with God, one another, and the rest of creation."[6] It does not take us long to observe the catastrophic results of sin in the story of Scripture and our own lives.

First, humanity's relationship of fellowship with God is broken. Then, humanity's relationship with one another is broken. Husband and wife will struggle against one another. Brothers will kill one another. Men will brag about their violence and sexual conquests. Eventually, nations will arise from the offspring of man and woman, and they will go to war with one another. Finally, the world that humanity was tasked to subdue and multiply in becomes a hostile environment. Animals that once lived peacefully among one another and humanity become wild. The very soil of the earth resists Adam's labor, fighting back, as it were, with thorns and barrenness. And death began its dark reign over all the inhabitants of the earth. Sin "wrecks human lives, and it leaves us broken and vulnerable."[7]

Whether you realized it or not, you have felt the impact of Adam and Eve's rebellion in your own life: conflict between persons is an obvious example. If you've ever had poison ivy, you know the fallen nature of creation!

So, while most people do not like to think about sin or be labeled a "sinner," most of those same people would admit that sin, however variously defined, is a universal reality. You might not like the word, but you perceive the presence of evil and brokenness in the world.

Almost everywhere we turn, we find sin and its impact on the world. Admittedly, we go through seasons when there is not much of a national conscience regarding sin, but occasionally we see glimpses of outrage over injustice that remind everyone that something is desperately wrong.

Take, for instance, the #MeToo movement. According to Pew Research, the term "MeToo" was coined in 2006 by activist Tarana Burke, but it became a viral movement in 2017 in the form of a hashtag on social media.[8] The movement rightly aimed to bring awareness to the reality of sexual harassment and assault. And while the public was not unanimous

If "right" and "wrong" are simply determined based on what the majority of humans in a particular society define instead of by God who made us to reflect Him, then how is it possible to say that things like abuse, murder, theft, corporate greed, or the dumping of toxic waste are "evil"?

in its support, most people appeared to decry sexual harassment and assault as morally wrong. The outrage was palpable. Yet, there were few public attempts to reconcile moral outrage with the deeply religious category of sin.

People knew that something was wrong. Sexual abuse was (and is) abhorrent. But few people seemed to wrestle with "why" it is wrong. If humanity has no ultimate purpose, no *telos*, if there is no immovable, inflexible, transcendent standard of justice and righteousness in the world, and if "right" and "wrong" are simply determined based on what the majority of humans in a particular society define at that time in history instead of by our relationship to God who made us to reflect Him, then how is it possible to say that things like abuse, murder, theft, corporate greed, or the dumping of toxic waste are "evil"? Surely there is a better way to make such a determination! Do we really want to live in a world where right and wrong are determined by those who perpetrate evil?

A Christian understanding of what's wrong in our world takes the judgment of sin out of the hands of sinners and places it back where it belongs: in the hands of an all-loving, all-knowing, all-powerful, all-righteous, and just God whose purpose for humanity is to glorify Him by reflecting Him, and ultimately, a plan to deal with all unrighteousness and injustice in the world.

For now, though, we need to see that our understanding of sin—of what's evil and wrong with the world—must come from God Himself. If it does not come from Him, then we are left with society having to come up with a consensus of what is right and wrong. And if you think that sounds like a good idea, I encourage you to read the book of Judges in the Old Testament. Trust me, you don't want to live in a world where "everyone does what is right in their own eyes" (see Judg. 21:25). But beyond this, we need to recognize that no one is more upset and displeased with sin in this world than the One who created this world with a specific purpose.

RECOGNIZING SIN

Just as our ability to recognize "the good" depends on God, our ability to recognize sin also depends on Him. Sin has resulted in all of humanity being born with a broken moral compass. We know intuitively that things are wrong, but we don't exactly understand why they are wrong. I saw this with my children as they grew up. I didn't have to teach them that stealing toys from each other in the church nursery was wrong. Somehow, they just knew that others should not steal from them. But they didn't really understand why that was the case. Even as they grew in maturity, not only did they experience being wronged by others, but they also wronged others themselves (something else that I didn't have to teach them). Most in our society continue to function with this innate sense of right and wrong, but when asked to explain "why" it is wrong, they are often left grasping for answers.

When we take what God has given us and use it for something contrary to His purpose, we desire it and use it for evil, and this is what God calls "sin."

When we do not consider God in our recognition of sin, we basically end up with something like a community consensus. For many, this sounds acceptable, until the community consensus turns against them. Just imagine, for a moment, how awful it would be to live in a neighborhood where the community consensus is that it is okay to steal from one another. The might of the majority doesn't make the will of the majority right or good. Just because a large group of people agree that something is right or something is wrong doesn't make it so. We need a transcendent standard outside of us to show us what is right and wrong. And that transcendent standard comes from God.

As we've discussed in the last chapter, God has made Himself known through two forms of revelation: general and special. And we know His general revelation is "very good." Yet, even with the goodness of general revelation, we need further revelation because of sin. While we can observe creation and discern aspects of good and evil, this does not change our hearts or lead us to conform our lives to God's will. This is one of the reasons why the apostle Paul speaks of sexual sins in Romans 1 as going against nature. We have the capacity to observe God's order in nature, but when we attempt to navigate life in creation with a broken moral compass, we turn good things into evil things.

Take, for instance, a tree. A tree can be used for all sorts of good things. It can be used to build shelter or a place of worship, but it can also be used to make idols or weapons to harm others. When God's creation is desired and used according to its created purpose, we use it for good. However, when we take what God has given us and use it for something contrary to His purpose, we desire it and use it for evil, and this is what God calls "sin." This is what we, by nature and choice, do apart from God's special revelation. God's special revelation corrects our evil desires and behaviors and directs them back to their created purpose. His special revelation corrects and transforms our moral compass so that we can navigate life in this world in a manner that honors God's purposes for His creation.

SIN AND DEATH IN THE SHADOW OF CHRIST

This chapter has contained its share of bad news, but I hope that you have a better understanding of the crisis that sin has created in us and our world. Rest assured: hope lies ahead! While sin led to crisis within creation, it is not as though the Creator was unaware or taken by surprise. As Romans 8:19–21 tells us, "Creation waits in eager expectation for the children of God to be revealed. For the creation was subjected to frustration, not by its own choice, but by the will of the one who subjected it, in hope that the creation itself will be liberated from its bondage to decay and brought into the freedom and glory of the children of God." Sin and the devastation that it has brought do not get the final word.

When we are navigating the world, we must give due attention to the fact that it is a broken world full of broken people in need of God's grace and mercy. If we do not adequately acknowledge the brokenness that sin has introduced into the world, we will misunderstand what is at stake and how to approach the world. So, let's conclude this segment by considering a few questions to help us discern how to reflect God and love others in our sexually broken world.

1. How does my approach to this situation acknowledge that we live in a world broken by sin? For instance, how is my understanding of who I am and how I am to live in this world informed by a true view of how sin has marred and broken so many things within me and in this present world?

2. How does my approach to this situation account for the real problem of sin? Does my view of myself and the world downplay the pervasiveness of sin? Or does it acknowledge what God's Word acknowledges about the corrupting impact of sin in my heart (Jer. 17:9)?

If we attempt to make sense of what we see in the world without acknowledging the brokenness by sin, we will be led astray. We will attempt to navigate this broken world with a broken compass. We need our minds to be renewed, which comes through Jesus Christ.

As we've begun to build a biblical and theological framework of God's good creation and what has gone wrong, let's next consider a couple of the practical issues people ask about our topic at hand: Is homosexuality in the Bible? and, Did Jesus speak about homosexuality?

CHAPTER THREE

Is Homosexuality Really in the Bible?— Bible Translations and Modern Language

People think all sorts of things are in the Bible that aren't really there. What kind of fruit did Adam and Eve eat in the garden of Eden? Growing up, I would have said it was an apple. But if you read the chapter on creation, you already know that there is no mention of an apple, just that it was fruit from a tree (Gen. 2:15–17). Somewhere along the way I was taught that it was an apple and just assumed that was the case, but I was wrong.

Or how about Jonah and the whale? Did you know that the text of Jonah only mentions a "great fish"? Nothing is said explicitly about the type of "great fish" in that story. While a whale may sound like a good candidate, though it's technically a mammal, if we go by the text itself, we must admit that we are not told what kind of creature swallowed him whole.

Or what about the proverb "Cleanliness is next to godliness"? Have you ever heard that one quoted before as if it was found in the Bible? I did, but again, it's not there. Or how about "Money is the root of all evil"? The Bible says something similar to this, but it does not say that money is the root of all evil, but rather that "the *love* of money is a root of *all kinds* of evil" (1 Tim. 6:10).

ABOUT THAT MANSION

Many people are acquainted with the King James Bible and its wording of well-known passages. One of these is John 14:2: "In my Father's house are many mansions: if it were not so, I would have told you." This verse has inspired all sorts of thoughts and reflections on heaven, and even songs. A "mansion" to look forward to sounds great, doesn't it?

Well, you can imagine how dismayed I was when I learned that the word that the King James Version had translated as "mansion" didn't mean what I had been taught it meant. It turns out that the way that the word "mansion" made its way into the Tyndale Bible and eventually the King James Version is from the Latin Vulgate, which translated the Greek word, *monē*, into the Latin word *mansiones*.[1] In Latin, the word *mansiones* and its Elizabethan English counterpart *mansions* meant "dwelling place, and not necessarily a palatial dwelling."[2]

Thus, almost all modern translations have opted to translate the Greek word *monē* as "dwelling place" or "rooms," which, if you think about it, makes a lot more sense considering that Jesus has just mentioned the "Father's house." But don't fret; we get something much better than a "mansion just over the hilltop," as one hymn writer put it. We get a permanent dwelling place in the presence of our heavenly Father!

This example of translation methods is an important reminder of the danger of imposing our ideas of words and concepts back onto the biblical text. Now, you may be asking, "What does a translation of John 14:2 have to do with our understanding of homosexuality?" As Christians, we need to have a better understanding of how Bible translation works, how it relates to modern language, and what that means for constructing a theological answer to important questions. There is a public conversation right now about whether or not Bible translators have gotten it right when they have used the word "homosexual" or "homosexuality" to translate certain ancient words. I will lay out the arguments that are being made and consider whether Christians should find such arguments to be compelling.

A MISTRANSLATION?

In the 2023 documentary titled *1946: The Mistranslation That Shifted Culture*, the writers argue that the release of the Revised Standard Version of the Bible in 1946 "mistranslated" *arsenokoitai* and *malakoi* as "homosexual" instead of representing the actual Greco-Roman background. As the argument goes, within the Greco-Roman world, *arsenokoitai* and *malakoi* were terms used to describe the active and passive male participants in the sexual act.

As most Bible scholars will admit, such an act was not restricted to people who only or exclusively engaged in this act. We know from ancient Greco-Roman literature that some men who had sex with their wives and other women in society also had sex with other men. The social dynamic at play in most of these sexual encounters was one of power or domination. Men of higher status within society would sexually engage other men of lower status not only for sexual pleasure but also to exert their dominance.

This documentary and several scholars conclude that these words— *arsenokoitai* and *malakoi*—are about power and oppression and are unrelated to homosexuality as it is now understood in society. Thus, they do not believe that these words should be understood or translated as referring to modern-day homosexual orientation or behaviors.

As a result, they argue that this is a mistranslation, which has resulted in trauma and oppression of same-sex-attracted individuals who want to live as Christians in committed, monogamous relationships with people of the same sex. In their eyes, neither the authors of the Bible nor the surrounding Greco-Roman culture had a category for "loving, committed same-sex relationships" or the idea of "homosexuality" as an orientation. And because these ancient writers supposedly did not possess these categories, these words should not be used in translation, just like the idea of "mansions" in John 14:2. Is such an explanation true?

Not every original text has a word that corresponds exactly to a word in a modern language. All translation work will involve some degree of discretion and decision by the translation committees.

HOW BIBLE TRANSLATION WORKS

Let's deal with some of the complexities that surround Bible translation. When a translator of any sort attempts to communicate a message from one language in a particular culture to another language in a different culture, they will typically adopt a philosophy of translation that falls somewhere on a spectrum.

Formal equivalent

On one end of the spectrum, you have a philosophy of translation that many refer to as a "formal equivalent." A translator operating from the formal equivalent perspective typically tries to produce a near word-for-word translation. These translators are concerned with preserving the "form" of the original text, even if that means it is more difficult for people to read. To give an example from the words mentioned above, a formal equivalent translation might translate the word *arsenokoitai* as "man-bedder." With the word *malakoi,* the formal equivalent would be something like passive or effeminate. One of the goals of such a translation is to limit the degree of interpretation that takes place in the work of translation.

When critical scholars say that entire generations of translation teams have "mistranslated" the Bible, we must be able to get into the weeds a little to see if the argument holds up. And to get into the weeds, we must know how Bible translation works. Not every original text has a word that corresponds exactly to a word in a modern language. All translation work will involve some degree of discretion and decision-making by the translation committees. It is as much an art as it is a science, which means we should be slow to accept the claim Bible translators have mistranslated something in our modern versions.

Dynamic equivalent

On the other side of the translation philosophy spectrum, we have what is called the "dynamic equivalent" perspective. With this translation approach, the translator aims to produce a more thought-for-thought translation of the original text. In other words, the translator will necessarily do some interpretation of the original text and then choose words in the new language that best fit with the thoughts being communicated by the original text. If a translator from a dynamic equivalent perspective were to translate the words *arsenokoitai* and *malakoi*, you would get something like "men who have sex with men," which simply combines these two words to make a statement.[3]

When Bible translators move from the ancient context of the Bible, they must make decisions about the degree to which a word or concept corresponds in our context to the words and concepts from the ancient context. This is how pretty much all translation works. So, do our modern translations of words like *arsenokoitai* and *malakoi* get it right when they translate these words as "homosexual"? Our answer to this question will largely depend on what we believe the Bible teaches or doesn't teach about the idea of sexual orientation.

SEXUAL ORIENTATION AND ANCIENT SOCIETIES

For the sake of the argument, let's consider the American Psychological Association's definition of sexual orientation: "An often enduring pattern of emotional, romantic, and/or sexual attractions to men, women, or both. [Sexual orientation] also refers to an individual's sense of personal and social identity based on those attractions, related behaviors, and membership in a community of others who share those attractions and behaviors."[4] To be clear, I'm presenting this definition for the sake of the argument, not because I necessarily agree with it or think that you should agree with it. Instead, I want us to deal honestly with the arguments that are being made by those who say that homosexuality as we understand it now did not exist in the era of the New Testament.

Part of what it means to love others well is to accurately understand what they are saying so that we can answer the actual questions they are asking instead of committing the "straw man fallacy," which basically means attacking a view that one's opponent doesn't actually hold or agree with. Maybe you have not heard this type of fallacious argument before, but trust me, it is out there. "Blue is a beautiful color." "Why do you hate red?" I most frequently encounter it on social media platforms like TikTok or Instagram, where today's teenagers spend a great deal of time.

As the argument typically goes, people will say that there is nothing within the era of the New Testament that even remotely approximates the idea of sexual orientation that we currently maintain within our society. What they mean by this is that there is nothing within the era of the New Testament that corresponds to the idea that some people may have experienced or were aware that people experienced "an often enduring pattern of emotional, romantic, and/or sexual attractions to men, women, or both" sexes. Instead, the argument is that biblical authors like the apostle Paul were primarily concerned with "excessive lust," or issues related to "abusive and exploitative sexual practices." Another way this has been stated is that "the ancient tradition of historic Christianity appears never to have had a moral category to describe homosexual persons."[5]

"[Some] have argued that since ancient moralists regarded homosexuality as a manifestation of an insatiable heterosexual lust and we do not, their opposition to homosexuality (including Paul's) must be disregarded in our own society."

Thus, the conclusion is that because these categories were not available or known at the time, the Bible could not have spoken to them.

Let's summarize these recent approaches that challenge the traditional view of historic Christianity. First, let's look at the argument that says that writers like the apostle Paul were concerned with "excessive lust" and not the concept of homosexuality as it is now understood. "[Some] have argued that since ancient moralists regarded homosexuality as a manifestation of an insatiable heterosexual lust and we do not, their opposition to homosexuality (including Paul's) must be disregarded in our own society."[6]

Certain scholars believe that the problem that biblical authors addressed was heterosexual people whose gratuitous lust or desires led them to have sex with people of the same sex.[7] In their view, the problem was excessive desire, not homosexuality in and of itself.

In terms of other arguments used to circumvent the traditional understanding of what the Bible teaches about homosexuality, we find some who argue that, given his seemingly cultural use of the words "nature" and "disgrace" regarding hair styles in 1 Corinthians 11:14, Paul is dealing with cultural expectations for men and women instead of referring to nature as part of the fixed created order.[8] Therefore, they conclude that what Paul teaches in Romans 1:26–27 is more about cultural issues that are subject to change over time and do not have any contemporary bearing on how we answer questions for people living in today's world.[9]

In fact, some, though not many, would argue that Paul's comment about "natural sexual relations" and "unnatural ones" in Romans 1:26–27 should be interpreted as speaking of heterosexual people who, "contrary to their heterosexual nature," engaged in homosexual acts.[10]

A final argument, which complements the first and which I have already briefly mentioned, is the idea that there is no evidence from this time period to suggest that people had any understanding that people might have an innate sexual attraction for someone of the same sex. Consider a few examples from popular books that argue for a revision of the traditional historic Christian understanding of sexuality. First, we have David Gushee's *Changing Our Mind*, in which he states, "The Church never had a category called 'sexual orientation' in its ancient tradition."[11] In a more roundabout but similar manner in *God and the Gay Christian*, Matthew Vines writes, "The modern understanding of homosexuality as a sexual orientation began to develop among an elite group of German psychiatrists in the late nineteenth century. Prior to 1869, terms meaning 'homosexual' and 'homosexuality' didn't exist in any language, and they weren't translated into English until 1892."[12]

If this argument were true, then we should not expect to find any examples within ancient literature of people who were innately attracted to others of the same sex. The biblical authors could not have possibly been expected to address moral issues related to people who were innately attracted to the same sex because, as the argument goes, we have no evidence of such people existing. Or, to be more straightforward, homosexuality wasn't a thing (as defined by the American Psychological Association) during the time of the New Testament.

But is this assumption true?

UNDERSTANDING ANCIENT SOURCES

In 1996, Bernadette Brooten wrote a watershed scholarly work titled *Love Between Women: Early Christian Responses to Female Homoeroticism*.[13] Brooten's work explored the relatively neglected topic of ancient perspectives on romantic relationships between women. Brooten demonstrates with painstaking attention to detail that the concept of homosexuality put forward by scholars who wish to overturn the traditional readings of Christianity on the topic of sexuality is misguided. While it may be true that many (although not all) ancient sources speak of male homoeroticism as either related to the oppressive practice of pederasty (sexual activity between an adult male and a youth) or the gratuitous lusts, this is not the case with female homoeroticism. In summarizing the findings of Brooten's book, Preston Sprinkle writes, "Brooten shows that some ancient writers believed that same-sex desires were fixed at birth. She gets this from looking at various medical, astrological, and magical texts."[14]

The evidence found in Brooten's book shows that it is misguided at best and wrong at worst to claim that there is no similarity between our modern conception of sexual orientation and what we find in the ancient sources about love between women. Consider how Brooten concludes her massive study on these ancient sources:

> This collection of ancient sources, never before examined together in one study, establishes the necessity for studying love between women on its own, rather than as a minor subcategory of male homoeroticism. Theories recently put forth by other scholars concerning sexual love between males in antiquity do not stand the test of these sources.[15]

What does this mean? It means that for decades scholars have either been unaware or intentionally ignoring evidence that suggests that some concept of sexual orientation was present in the ancient sources. And in case you are wondering if Brooten's conclusions mean she is sympathetic to the traditional Christian interpretation of these passages that deal with sexuality, let me assure you, she is not. Brooten writes in an attempt to liberate homoeroticism from the moral constraints of historic Christianity. She disagrees with the apostle Paul's understanding of sexuality, but at least she is willing to interpret Paul in his ancient context instead of trying to reinterpret him in light of our present context.

Brooten's work undermines the assumption that the idea of sexual orientation, however underdeveloped it may have been in ancient times, was not available or known during the time of the New Testament or the early church. Or, to put it another way, what we understand to be "homosexuality" now is not entirely unlike the ideas of sexuality that are present in the ancient sources.

TERMS AND CATEGORIES

When scholars say concepts like "sexual orientation" were unknown to the biblical authors and thus their works do not address the issues inherent in such a modern concept, they are making generalizations that are not actually supported by the ancient evidence. For instance, when David Gushee states that the "church never had a category called 'sexual orientation' in its ancient tradition," or Matthew Vines tells us that the terms "homosexual" or "homosexuality" didn't exist until the nineteenth century, the implication is that no one could have possibly identified the ideas contained within those categories or terms before the modern era. Yet, as Brooten's work shows, there is evidence of an awareness in ancient times of people experiencing "enduring patterns of emotional, romantic, and/or sexual attractions to men, women, or both" sexes.

Ancient writers didn't have to use specific terms that were developed later in history to describe what they observed or experienced in their own lives or the lives of other people. This is typically how historical and sociological study works. Historians and social scientists reflect on what ancient people wrote, said, and did, then analyze and label it with categories and terms. Surely that does not mean that by labeling something, they have created it, does it?

In light of this, I don't think we need to be afraid of using familiar or even modern language to describe what we find in ancient sources if it can be demonstrated that the words we are using fit what we actually see in those sources and have "some overlap, some semblance" to our modern concepts.[16] As Brooten's work shows, there may be some differences (as we would naturally expect) between our modern conception of sexual orientation and ancient understandings of sexuality, but human sexuality and the experiences it often entails are not entirely unique or different over the course of history. This is true not only of sexuality, but of life and language in general, which is important to remember, given what we will consider about translations in the next section.

We've got to be willing to listen and learn as we work to love others well. This means avoiding caricatures of people and the positions that they hold.

MODERN TRANSLATIONS AND HOMOSEXUALITY

If the section above teaches us anything, I hope that it teaches us that if we are going to offer thoughtful answers to sincere questions, we've got to be willing to listen and learn as we work to love others well. This means avoiding caricatures of people and the positions that they hold. No one wants to be misunderstood, so as an act of love toward others, let's prioritize speaking truthfully, even as we engage with positions that do not represent our own.

So, what about the question that we started this chapter with—if "homosexuality" is even addressed in the Bible. I began this chapter by considering two Greek words: *arsenokoitai* and *malakoi*. While the first word, *arsenokoitai*, is only used in two places in the New Testament (1 Cor. 6:9; 1 Tim. 1:10), both words are only used together in 1 Corinthians 6:9 to denote the active and passive participants in the sexual act. Thus, I'm going to primarily focus on 1 Corinthians 6:9 in this section. Let's consider how various translations have attempted to render this pair of words.

In the New International Version, 1 Corinthians 6:9 reads, "Or do you not know that wrongdoers will not inherit the kingdom of God? Do not be deceived: Neither the sexually immoral nor idolaters nor adulterers nor men who have sex with men." The phrase "men who have sex with men" attempts to give a sense of what these two terms might mean together.

By way of contrast, in the New American Standard Bible (NASB 1995), 1 Corinthians 6:9 reads, "Or do you not know that the unrighteous will not inherit the kingdom of God? Do not be deceived; neither fornicators, nor idolaters, nor adulterers, nor effeminate, nor homosexuals." With the NASB 1995 translation, we see the translator using the word "effeminate" to render *malakoi*, and the word "homosexual" to render *arsenokotai*. This is a slightly more literal rendering of the two words, though the translators do opt to use the word "homosexual" to denote the active partner in the sexual act while separating the word "effeminate" from the act itself. The reason(s) translators of the NASB might have chosen to separate the words in this verse is left for the reader. It may be that they intended to allow the word "effeminate" to stand on its own so that Paul could address "male prostitutes," most likely engaged in ritual sex in the local temples. Or it may simply be because of the translators' commitment to a more formal translation theory.

To give you another example, consider how the English Standard

Version renders 1 Corinthians 6:9: "Or do you not know that the unrighteous will not inherit the kingdom of God? Do not be deceived: neither the sexually immoral, nor idolaters, nor adulterers, nor men who practice homosexuality." Here we find something of a middle road between the NIV 2011 and the NASB 1995. Whereas the NIV 2011 states, "men who have sex with men," the ESV categorizes that sexual act as "homosexuality." Then, whereas the NASB separates the "effeminate" from the "homosexual," the ESV combines the men addressed here and defines their act as the "practice of homosexuality." Given these different, nuanced renderings, let's look at the words themselves.

For the nerds out there (like me) who like to do their own word studies, *arsenokoitai* is the plural form of *arsenokoites*. As I mentioned earlier, this is a compound word that combines Greek words for "man" and "bed." Translated rigidly, it would mean something like "man-bedder." Obviously, the emphasis here is on the action, and not necessarily on "desire" or "attraction." This differentiation between action and attraction is part of the big debate on whether or not translators should use the words "homosexuality" or "homosexual" to render the terms *arsenokotai* and *malakoi*.

Several scholars note that the apostle Paul is likely drawing on Leviticus 18:22 and 20:13 from the Septuagint, a Greek translation of the Old Testament, when he uses the word *arsenokotai*.[17] In Leviticus 18:22, we read, "Do not have sexual relations with a man as one does with a woman; that is detestable." Leviticus 20:13 essentially restates the prohibition with its legal penalty when such an act was found to be committed in the land. In the Septuagint translation of Leviticus 18:22, the words *arsenos* and *koitēn* are used in the same phrase, but they are separated by the phrase *ou koimēthēsē*, which means "do not sleep with." In Leviticus 20:13, the words are found next to one another, but not in the compound form that we find in 1 Corinthians 6:9. The idea here is that men should not "sleep with" or "have sexual intercourse with" another man as they would with a woman, for such an act is "hated by God."[18] If Paul is drawing on Leviticus 18:22 and 20:13 in his use of *arsenokotai* in 1 Corinthians 6:9, then it becomes more obvious that he regards this prohibition against same-sex behavior from the Old Testament as an abiding ethic for God's kingdom people.

Paul is drawing upon his understanding of God's ideal for sexual relations as revealed in creation and taught in God's Word.

The Old Testament context of Leviticus 18:22 and 20:13 is broader in its prohibitions than the Greco-Roman context in which Paul wrote 1 Corinthians 6:9. Some have attempted to make 1 Corinthians 6:9 only about a limited expression of same-sex behavior (pederasty). This might make sense if Paul were only drawing from his surrounding culture, but if the use of the term *arsenokotai* likely arises from Leviticus 18:22 and 20:13, then we should not limit the meaning of 1 Corinthians 6:9 to mere categories present in the Greco-Roman context. Instead, we should interpret Paul within the context of his own Jewish, theological background, which would have been significantly formed and informed by the Old Testament.[19]

Paul is not just dealing with a narrow situation in Corinth when he uses the terms *arsenokotai* and *malakoi*. He is drawing upon his understanding of God's ideal for sexual relations as revealed in creation and taught in God's Word. Given what we understand about the Old Testament context that Paul draws upon, we should affirm that God's Word prohibits all same-sex behavior.

AN ART, NOT A SCIENCE

At the heart of many debates regarding the use of the terms "homosexual" or "homosexuality" in modern Bible translations is the idea that using such terms does not give due attention to the role of desire or innate erotic orientation. One might say, "Okay, the Bible is clear that same-sex behaviors are prohibited. They are outside of God's will for humanity."

But what about people who describe their sexuality as being oriented to a person of the same sex? If those scenarios are not necessarily in view in passages like 1 Corinthians 6:9, which are more about same-sex behaviors than desires, then why use a term like "homosexual" or "homosexuality" in those verses?

This is a fair question. As I have already mentioned, Bible translation is often as much an art as it is a science. Translators do not have an easy job. They are attempting to take ancient words and concepts and make them understandable to an audience far removed from the original context. Furthermore, it is not as if modern language remains static. Things change. If you don't believe me, just sit down and have a conversation with a teenager and listen to the way they speak. Just the other day, I heard one of my kids describe their sibling as "pressed." This means something like "stressed out," "frustrated," or "mad." Anyway, in time, if the word "pressed" gets used enough in this way, the new definition will eventually make it into the dictionary. It could be that thirty years from now, it will be commonplace to understand the word "pressed" in this way. And if that is the case, don't be surprised to find the word used in a future translation of the Bible. That's just how language works.

I share this because I think that what has happened in society with the use of the words "homosexual" and "homosexuality" is that the definitions of these terms have continued to shift and expand over time. In the case of these two terms, we have observed a shift from a focus on behavior to a focus on innate desire. What those terms meant when the NASB was being translated back in 1977 and 1995 likely do not mean the exact same thing that they mean now. This means we shouldn't ascribe ill intent to the translators of the NASB but rather understand that language shifts and expands and that Bible translators will constantly be working to update their translations to be as clear as possible for their audiences in the future. And I believe we are already seeing that take place with Bible translations.

Just consider how the Holman Christian Standard Bible, which was originally translated in 1999, recently updated its translation of 1 Corinthians 6:9 with its new edition, the Christian Standard Bible, in 2017.[20] The 1999 version translated *arsenokoitai* and *malakoi* as "anyone practicing homosexuality." But in the 2017 version, these terms were translated as "males who have sex with males." The more recent translation seems to have taken into consideration the fact that the term "homosexuality" is somewhat of a moving target, always subject to redefinition and expansion.

It's probably best to retire the term "homosexuals" or "homosexuality" as a modern translation of the words arsenokoitai and malakoi, since our society's understanding of those terms appears to be constantly in flux.

So, instead of using the term "homosexuality," the translators opted for a more literal rendering, "males who have sex with males."

Is this a compromise? Some may say that it is, but I do not think so. Instead, I think it is an attempt at providing greater clarity in keeping with the language Paul used in the passage and trying to anticipate that linguistic baggage that a modern audience might bring to their reading of the text. To that end, it's probably best to retire the term "homosexuals" or "homosexuality" as a modern translation of the words *arsenokoitai* and *malakoi*, since our society's understanding (or misunderstanding) of those terms appears to be constantly in flux. This, however, is not to say that we have "no idea" what *arsenokoitai* or *malakoi* meant in their original context. Paul, in no uncertain terms, believed and taught that same-sex sexual relations were contrary to God's will for His creation.

Most Bible translation committees are doing their best to honor the biblical authors' intention by using the best terms and ideas that they have available to them at the time to communicate ancient truths to a modern audience. This is just like the example in John 14:2, where we have seen modern translation update the language because the word "mansions" has shifted in its meaning. As the vocabulary of modern audiences shifts, Bible translators will have to keep working hard to produce intelligible versions of the Bible.

SO, IS HOMOSEXUALITY REALLY IN THE BIBLE?

We are back where we started with our question, "Is homosexuality really in the Bible?" I know it has been a circuitous route to get to this point but thank you for your patience. One might conclude from the previous section that because the word "homosexual" is probably not the best term to use to translate the Greek words found in 1 Corinthians 6:9, the answer to the question would be a resounding "no." Such an answer, however, does not take into consideration how Christians have historically "done theology." Constructing a theology of what the Bible teaches about sexuality requires far more than simply looking at a few Bible verses where certain terms are used.

For instance, one of the most important passages in all of Scripture for understanding biblical sexuality is Romans 1:24–27. Consider what Paul writes to the church in Rome,

> Therefore God gave them over in the sinful desires of their hearts to sexual impurity for the degrading of their bodies with one another. They exchanged the truth about God for a lie, and worshiped and served created things rather than the Creator— who is forever praised. Amen.
>
> Because of this, God gave them over to shameful lusts. Even their women exchanged natural sexual relations for unnatural ones. In the same way the men also abandoned natural relations with women and were inflamed with lust for one another. Men committed shameful acts with other men, and received in themselves the due penalty for their error.

Notice what Paul says and does not say in this passage. First, he does not draw a distinction between lustful desire and behavior, as if one was neutral and the other was sinful. Both the desire and the behavior are regarded as sinful. Yet, unlike in 1 Corinthians 6:9 and 1 Timothy 1:10, Paul does not use the terms *arsenokoitai* or *malakoi*. Instead, as many scholars understand this passage—and I agree—Paul describes what is happening when people abandon God's design for sex. When people desire and engage in unnatural sexual behaviors, which is best understood as abandoning God's design for the male-female sexual relationship, they are guilty before God for exchanging the truth that He has embedded within our bodies and revealed in His Word for a lie.

At the core of this lie is the deceptive belief that God as Creator has no say over what is right for His creation to think or how His creation is to behave. If this sounds familiar, it's because it is. This is very similar to what we considered in the chapters on creation and crisis, where Adam and Eve did not trust that God's design for them was right or the best. And as we saw there, such a refusal to trust God and His design has devastating consequences.

So, when Paul highlights the exchange of the natural for the unnatural, we should see God's created order as providing a normative ethic for His creation. When that created order is violated, the violation is regarded as unnatural. In Romans 1:24–27, Paul points to homosexuality as an example of violating God's created order by exchanging the natural order of male-female sexual relations for the unnatural order of same-sex sexual relations. As such, Paul unequivocally condemns these relations, and it's not just traditional scholars who acknowledge this understanding of Romans 1:24–27. Consider, again, Bernadette Brooten's comments on these verses:

> Paul could have believed that *tribades* [the active female partners in a female homosexual bond], the ancient *kinaidoi* [the passive male partners in a male homosexual bond] and other sexually unorthodox persons were born that way and yet still condemn them as unnatural and shameful. . . . I believe that Paul used the word "exchanged" to indicate that people knew the natural sexual order of the universe and left it behind. . . . I see Paul as condemning all forms of homoeroticism as the unnatural acts of people who had turned away from God.[21]

Any endeavor to sanctify same-sex sexual relations from the Bible is simply disingenuous to the evidence. "The idea that homosexuals might be redeemed by mutual devotion would have been wholly foreign to Paul or any Jew or early Christian."[22] The most honest approach to this question would be for revisionist theologians and ethicists to admit that their attempt to normalize and solemnize same-sex relations in the Christian community cannot be sustained or supported by Scripture.

More certainly could be and has been written about Romans 1:24–27, but I mention it here to show the importance of how we attempt to answer questions about what the Bible teaches on a topic.

Without ever using the terms that are often a key focus in the whole modern debate about homosexuality in the Bible, we know that, as did all Jews and the Jewish believers in his time, Paul condemned homosexual behavior. Limiting the conversation to issues about translation is simply too narrow and leads to biased results.

God's Word addresses our actions and our thoughts, both of which are submitted to the scrutiny of the holy wisdom of our all-knowing God.

As a rule, Christians do not formulate the teachings (doctrines) of God's Word based solely on one or two verses. So, instead of looking simply at a passage like 1 Corinthians 6:9 and concluding that because the passage deals with behavior more than desire, "the Bible must not have anything to say about what we understand about homosexuality now," we have to move beyond the question of Bible translations and consider what the whole of Scripture teaches us about God's will for both our sexual behaviors and desires.

To answer the question of whether homosexuality, as it is currently understood in society, is in the Bible requires us to expand our vision of how the Scripture addresses each aspect mentioned in the APA's definition. As we will see in later chapters, God's Word addresses our actions and our thoughts, both of which are submitted to the scrutiny of the holy wisdom of our all-knowing God. We must give greater attention to all that Scripture teaches about sexuality, our desires, and our identity in Christ. Understanding what Scripture teaches about these things is not simply a matter of picking the right words when moving from one cultural setting to the next. We must allow the totality of God's Word to inform our understanding of His will for our lives as followers of Christ.

Discerning what the Bible teaches about homosexuality is much like discerning the Bible's teaching on the doctrine of the Trinity. We do not simply look at one or two verses and expect those verses to explain every detail about what Scripture teaches about the triune nature of God. Instead, we give attention to the whole testimony of Scripture on the topic and, from there, construct the doctrine of the Trinity. Similarly, in discerning the Bible's teaching on homosexuality, we need to pay attention to how all of Scripture speaks to how we are to live, especially when it comes to our sexuality as a people who God has created for His holy purpose.

What feels like condemnation can actually result in leading us to freedom.

WHERE'S THE LOVE?

I am aware of how this chapter may feel to those who may already know these things and are chiefly concerned with how to live out the things they know among their friends and family.

Since this book is addressing practicalities from a theological framework, there are a few reasons why I wanted to consider this question early on. First, I can't assume that everyone is aware of everything covered in this chapter. Second, some of the concerns that readers have are in how to address what revisionist theologians and ethicists are teaching.

Accessing teaching once required a person to purchase a book or attend a seminar, but now all kinds of information is freely available on all sorts of online platforms. You might be surprised to know how often I see these types of revisionist arguments on popular social media platforms, especially among those who have labeled themselves as "deconstructing Christians" or "exvangelicals." I wanted to help those trying to help others wrestle with big questions like the one in this chapter.

I also want you to understand that I am a firm believer in the power of God's Word, working through the Holy Spirit to set people free from sin by bringing them to faith in Christ. The point of speaking so candidly about sin is not to bury people in inescapable guilt or ostracize them because of their struggle but to demonstrate their need for the Savior. Our God is the God who is described as being "rich in mercy," who saves us not based on our performance but based on His grace toward us in Jesus Christ (Eph. 2:1–10). If we had no awareness of our sin and our need of the Savior, we would never know the grace of God.

So, please hear me, because "God demonstrates his own love for us in this: While we were still sinners, Christ died for us" (Rom. 5:8). We should love sinners, being aware of our own sin, knowing that talking about it and telling others is not an act of hate, but love, even if those who initially hear it do not perceive it at the time. Don't allow the culture's definition of what it means to be loving keep you from actually loving others in the truth. As Paul taught us in 1 Corinthians 13:6, "Love does not delight in evil but rejoices with the truth."

CHAPTER FOUR

"Jesus Never Spoke About Homosexuality"

A s a pastor, I hear some wild things. It just comes with the territory.

I could fill volumes with some of the things I've come across, but I'll just give you one. I was speaking with a congregant one day when he said something startling.

"My father spoke to me," he said.

"Your—oh, I'm sorry, I thought your father was deceased," I replied.

"He is, he is," the man answered. "He spoke from beyond the grave with a message for me. He told me it was fine for me to divorce my wife! Boy, am I ever glad. I'll be sure to honor his wishes."

Now, I had an excellent seminary education. However, I never had a course on counseling a necromancer!

This, and thankfully less extreme experiences, taught me that I had to learn how to adapt my approach to interpreting and applying the Bible to each pastoral situation that I encountered because many of the questions and comments that I would field from congregants would be new and fresh.[1] Comments like the situation mentioned above can stretch us. And that was precisely the case when I encountered the claim that we are dealing with in this chapter.

DID JESUS EVER SPEAK ABOUT HOMOSEXUALITY?

"But Jesus never spoke about homosexuality." You may have heard or seen this objection raised more than once. At first glance, such an argument appears legitimate. A simple word search online or a perusal of a Bible concordance reveals that the words "homosexual" or "homosexuality" are not found on Jesus' lips. The idea here is that because Jesus never said anything specifically about homosexuality, then we would do well to follow His lead. Open and shut case, right?

An often-quoted axiom states: "The absence of evidence is not evidence of absence."

Upon further consideration, though, we will find that this type of argument is fundamentally flawed. It is not right to assume that because we do not initially see or perceive evidence for a claim, we can conclude that no such evidence exists at all. When someone claims, "Jesus never spoke about homosexuality," the assumption is that Jesus held no beliefs or convictions about homosexuality. Such an assumption fails on at least two points.

First, the assumption that Jesus held no beliefs or convictions about homosexuality because there is no written record of Jesus speaking about these issues in Scripture fails to understand the nature of Scripture. Let me explain. The Scriptures record quite a bit of information about Jesus' life and ministry, but the Scriptures were not written as a comprehensive statement that contains every detail of every word or deed that Jesus spoke or performed. In fact, we are told the exact opposite. In John 21:25, we read, "Jesus did many other things as well. If every one of them were written down, I suppose that even the whole world would not have room for the books that would be written." To be sure, the author is employing exaggeration as a form of speech to make a point about Jesus' life and ministry, but even within this statement, we see that the gospel accounts were written and crafted for a specific purpose. They were not written to be exhaustive accounts but to communicate essential truths about Jesus so that different audiences would trust Jesus as Lord and Savior.

When people claim that "Jesus never spoke about homosexuality," they fail to reckon with the Jewishness of Jesus.

Thus, to conclude that Jesus "never spoke about homosexuality" requires the gospel accounts to be something that their authors never intended them to be, namely, exhaustive records of everything Jesus said or did before His ascension. If we wish to be fair to the gospel writers, then we should respect their intentions. Isn't that what we would expect from others with our own words?

Just because there is no explicit record of Jesus addressing homosexuality in the Scriptures, that does not mean that we can claim with certainty that "Jesus never spoke about homosexuality." It would be more accurate to say that the gospel writers recorded nothing about Jesus speaking on homosexuality. But does this mean that we cannot know anything about Jesus' view of sexuality? This is where we come to the second place, where the assumption about Jesus' apparent silence fails again.

When people claim that "Jesus never spoke about homosexuality," they fail to reckon with the Jewishness of Jesus. Jesus knew the Jewish

Scriptures and was more than pleased to affirm their truthfulness and authority for understanding God's will for His people. We frequently see Jesus asking those He encountered, "Have you not read?" which is often followed by some portion of Scripture from the Old Testament. How could Jesus ask such a question and then quote from Scripture if He did not affirm those passages as authoritative truth?

A careful reader of the Gospels will notice how often Jesus uses Scripture and draws upon all the sections of the Old Testament, which are referred to by the shorthand expression "the Law and the Prophets." And when He does so, He affirms them. Even when Jesus is teaching in the Sermon on the Mount (Matt. 5–7) and says things like, "You have heard it said . . . but I say to you," He is not questioning the truthfulness or authority of those passages, but instead was critiquing the way those passages had been understood and applied. And if this is the case, then we should be very slow to take the claim that "Jesus never spoke about homosexuality" as evidence that Jesus didn't have an opinion about human sexuality.

JESUS' BIBLE

If we are going to come to any conclusions about Jesus' perspective on homosexuality, then we need to deal seriously with the sources that Jesus regularly appealed to in life and ministry. I believe there are two significant points that we can make about Jesus and His Bible.

First, Jesus affirmed the Old Testament as God's Word. He treated the Old Testament as true. I could give example after example of this. Consider the people Jesus mentioned in His teaching, which demonstrates that He understood them to be historical people: Abel, Abraham, Moses, and Jonah (see Luke 11:51; John 8:56; Matt. 8:4; and

Matt. 12:39–41). In each case, Jesus assumes that these are historical people of whom the Old Testament speaks truthfully.

Jesus also affirmed the Old Testament as God's Word by appealing to the Old Testament as authoritative. When Jesus had a conflict with the Pharisees and scribes (Matt. 23:2–3; John 5:39–47) and the Sadducees (Matt. 22:31–32), He appealed to the Jewish Scriptures. Doing so demonstrates that Jesus, even as God in the flesh, held that the Old Testament was true and authoritative.

Finally, Jesus regarded the Old Testament as inspired. To speak of the Old Testament as "inspired" is to speak of it as originating with God Himself. The language of "inspired" can be misleading, given that we sometimes use it to describe an artistic impulse, like "the sunset inspired my painting," but that is not what I have in mind here. To speak of "inspiration" is to speak of Scripture as being "breathed out by God." Scripture has its origin in God Himself. Jesus taught this. We can see this in passages like Matthew 19:4–5, which quotes from Genesis 2:24. In Matthew 19:4–5, Jesus attributes the words of the author of Genesis to "the Creator." The intention here is not to undermine the role that Moses played as the author but rather to show that it is possible to speak both of "Scripture speaking" and "God speaking" in a way that is synonymous. I love the way that New Testament scholar John Wenham puts it: "What Scripture says is the Word of God—God is its author."[2] But why is this important? It is important because the Bible that Jesus affirmed as true, authoritative, and inspired also makes exceedingly clear statements about homosexuality.

JESUS AND THE OLD TESTAMENT
ON SEXUALITY AND MARRIAGE

Matthew 5:27–30

If I told you that someone would be waiting outside of your home tomorrow morning to destroy you, how would that impact or influence your morning routine? I bet that you would radically reorganize your day. You would live with an increased vigilance. This is how Jesus wants us to live every day, because there really is a threat lurking, trying to destroy us. Let's see how Jesus speaks about it in Matthew 5:27–30, where we read,

> "You have heard that it was said, 'You shall not commit adultery.' But I tell you that anyone who looks at a woman lustfully has already committed adultery with her in his heart. If your right eye causes you to stumble, gouge it out and throw it away. It is better for you to lose one part of your body than for your whole body to be thrown into hell. And if your right hand causes you to stumble, cut it off and throw it away. It is better for you to lose one part of your body than for your whole body to go into hell."

In this passage, Jesus draws attention to the things that we have heard from others. In this case, we have heard, "You shall not commit adultery." Found in Exodus 20:14, this is the seventh of the Ten Commandments. In Jesus' day, the religious leaders believed that they were keeping the commandments because they practiced an outward obedience, but they lacked an inward transformation. So, what does Jesus do? He redirects the people to the matter of the heart. Jesus is not concerned only with our outward behavior. He desires for us to have a pure heart, out of which obedience will spring.

In verse 28, Jesus goes to the heart of the issues, which is always the issue of the heart. While the religious leaders in His day were faithful in their outward obedience, they lacked inward transformation. What does this mean to "look at someone lustfully"? In the case of Matthew 5:28, this means to look at someone with a sexual desire or longing that is not in accordance with God's plan for sex. God's plan for sex is for it to be enjoyed between one man and one woman in the context of a monogamous marriage for a lifetime. Thus, Jesus is not speaking about all sexual desire, but rather, all sexual desire that violates God's intention for sex in the context of marriage.

In the case of the particular religious leaders in this passage, they were most likely not committing the physical act of adultery, but it does appear that they were desiring to do so in their heart. They were, as the Tenth Commandment states, coveting their neighbor's wife, which God explicitly forbids. In God's eyes, these religious leaders were guilty of adultery of the heart, which, while different from the actual act of adultery, still rendered these people guilty before God.

I'm sure all of us would admit to this same tendency. We tend to believe that we are not guilty before God because we have managed to avoid outward expressions of our inward lusts, but, according to Jesus, when we covet or desire that which God forbids, we are rendered guilty before a holy God. We are adulterers from the heart. So, how does Jesus deal with adulterers?

While He certainly hates the sin of adultery, He also welcomes and forgives those who come to Him in humility, seeking forgiveness and reconciliation. We see this in the story of Jesus and the woman caught in adultery, recounted in John 8:2–11.[3]

When the woman was brought before Jesus by the religious leaders for judgment, He rebukes the religious people for their self-righteous judgment. Then, He forgives and restores the woman, telling her to "Go now and leave your life of sin." In other words, Jesus forgives her, restores her, and then sanctifies her for holy living. He does not forgive her so that she can go on living in adultery. Instead, Jesus forgives her so that she might be set free from adultery to pursue holiness, to no longer live in sexual immorality, which is Jesus' aim in Matthew 5:27–30.

This brings us to verses 29–30, which are some of the most shocking verses in all of Scripture. In these two verses, Jesus intends to stir up our concern for holy living. He is calling the people to obey God. To do whatever is necessary to abandon actions and attitudes that do not conform to God's will for our lives. Yes. It is true that Jesus welcomes the adulterer. Yes. It is true that Jesus forgives the adulterer. Yes. It is true that Jesus gives new life. But we must say more! Jesus also calls the adulterer to holiness—to a radical pursuit of embodying the new life that He has given us!

These two graphic images of cut-off hands and gouged-out eyes are intended by Jesus to stir us up to see how vital it is for us to pursue holiness. As Grant Osborne said about this passage, "The two parallel metaphors mean simply that one must violently throw away everything that causes the lust, lest their spiritual life and ultimately their eternal destiny be destroyed in the process."[4] The point was not that cutting off hands or gouging out eyes would actually solve the problem of our sin, but rather, if such extreme measures would deal with our sins, then we should avail ourselves of them. We should care so much about holiness that we would take any measure necessary to deal with it.

Jesus wants us to see that there really is a threat waiting for us, waiting to destroy us, and that thing is called "sinful desire." For some, that may be sexual desire, for others, it may be another form of desire, but everyone is threatened. The enemy of our souls is walking around like a roaring lion, seeking to devour us. Jesus died to set us free from sin. Therefore, by His grace and mercy, we ought to take extreme measures to deal with sin in our lives, and this includes our sexual desires that are not in accordance with God's design for sin.

MATTHEW 5:31–32

Immediately following His warning against lust, Jesus turns His attention to the matter of faithfulness in marriage in verses 31–32, which state,

> "It has been said, 'Anyone who divorces his wife must give her a certificate of divorce.' But I tell you that anyone who divorces his wife, except for sexual immorality, makes her the victim of adultery, and anyone who marries a divorced woman commits adultery."

In these verses, Jesus corrects a misunderstanding and misapplication of Deuteronomy 24:1–4, which allowed people to get a divorce under specific, limited circumstances, such as the husband's finding "something indecent" about his wife. Scholars in Jesus' day debated what that meant. One school of thought was that a wife who spoiled the supper could be divorced. Another opined that a man who found a prettier woman could sever his marriage. The point was that Moses' words were misapplied to allow divorce for superficial reasons.

Thus, what Jesus is doing in verses 31–32 is returning to Moses' original intention in Deuteronomy 24:1, which was to protect the woman from a husband who might simply discard her without cause. That way her legal status would be as a legitimately divorced woman.

She would be protected from accusation of being an adulteress who violated her marriage or accused of living as a prostitute.

So, while divorce was not God's intention for marriage (as we will see below in Matthew 19), because of the hardness of man's heart, God made provision for protection by allowing divorce to formalize the separation of a husband and wife when the ground of the divorce was biblically justifiable.

In the case of Matthew 5, Jesus states that the ground is sexual immorality. Other portions of the New Testament, specifically 1 Corinthians 7, expounded upon the grounds for divorce to include abandonment, which I believe would also include abuse. Taken together, Jesus' instruction on marriage and divorce in Matthew 5 is a denunciation of the flippant way that the religious leaders of His day walked in and out of marriage without regard for its sanctity and purpose.

It is important to realize that while it is true that "God hates divorce," Scripture does not say that "God hates divorcees."

Why is marriage so important to God? Paul tells us in Ephesians 5 that it is because God intended for marriage to point us to the relationship of Christ and His church. Christ loves His church like a bride. Christ lays down His life for His bride. Christ sacrifices for and serves His bride. In response to Christ's love and service, the church should submit to Him and seek to honor Him. Yet, though Christ is always faithful, the church is not always faithful. But what does Christ do with His unruly bride? He does not abandon her. He does not abuse her. He does not divorce her. He is committed to her. He pursues her. He loves her. Like Hosea and Gomer in the Old Testament, Jesus comes after His rebellious bride with lovingkindness.

Jesus' example with the church is a far cry from the way the Pharisees and many in our culture view marriage and divorce. Instead of looking to our culture and our coworkers, we ought to look to the faithfulness that God has demonstrated toward us in Christ and seek to emulate that in our own marriages. God calls us to a faithfulness that confounds the conventional wisdom of our day.

It is important to realize that while it is true that "God hates divorce," Scripture does not say that "God hates divorcees." In fact, I believe that if you were to ask many people who have gone through divorce, they would say that they "hate divorce" too. Divorce, like death, was not part of God's original design for marriage. Divorce was granted as a concession to a sinful society so that people would not be vulnerable or preyed upon by others. So, while we must affirm what God's Word teaches about divorce, we also need to affirm God's love for those who have gone through the tragedy of divorce, or who are even a guilty party in their divorce. Life in a sinful world with relationships between sinful people does not always go as we would hope. Yet, in Christ, there is forgiveness offered to all who would call upon Him in faith.

God intends for our marriages to point to His faithfulness. When people see faithfulness in marriage, it should be a reminder of how God keeps His promises to His people. Furthermore, by inference, Jesus' teaching on marriage and divorce affirms the pattern of marriage that was revealed in creation. Marriage, in God's design, is a monogamous, covenantal relationship between one man and one woman for a lifetime.

MATTHEW 19:1–12

This passage draws our attention back to the creation account in Genesis 1–2, which reveals God's design for human sexuality. Let's revisit Genesis 1:26–28:

Then God said, "Let us make mankind in our image, in our likeness, so that they may rule over the fish in the sea and the birds in the sky, over the livestock and all the wild animals, and over all the creatures that move along the ground." So God created mankind in his own image, in the image of God he created them; male and female he created them. God blessed them and said to them, "Be fruitful and increase in number; fill the earth and subdue it. Rule over the fish in the sea and the birds in the sky and over every living creature that moves on the ground."

Immediately, we notice the creation of male and female, who are described as bearing God's image. As image bearers, they are responsible to rule over creation and increase in number. This is the creation mandate for male and female.

In Genesis 2:4–25, we see an expanded narrative about this relationship between male and female. The male, referred to here as "man," was formed by God from the dust and given life. The man was placed in the garden of Eden, but there was no suitable helper found among the rest of creation for man. So, God created a woman, the "female" from Genesis 1, as a companion for man for fulfilling the creation mandate. According to Genesis 2:23, the man said, "This is now bone of my bones and flesh of my flesh; she shall be called 'woman,' for she was taken out of man." Then, we are told in verses 24–26, "That is why a man leaves his father and mother and is united to his wife, and they become one flesh. Adam and his wife were both naked, and they felt no shame."

From the beginning, God revealed that His design for human sexuality was one man and one woman, joined together in marriage to rule over creation and increase in number through procreation. This was and is God's design for our sexuality. And Jesus affirmed this design for sexuality when He answered the Pharisees' question about divorce in Matthew 19:1–12. A marriage between one man and one woman is the context in which God designed humans to fulfill His purpose for sexuality. Except in situations where the marriage commitment had been broken (Matt. 19:8–9), God did not permit divorce. Marriage was to be a lifelong covenant commitment between one man and one woman with the aim of bearing and raising children as they ruled their respective spheres of creation.

> *God's ideal for marriage is between one man and one woman for a lifetime. This ideal excludes the possibility of any other arrangement falling within God's boundaries for marriage.*

According to Matthew 19:10, "The disciples said to him, 'If this is the situation between a husband and wife, it is better not to marry.'" In other words, to the disciples, such a commitment to sexual exclusivity in the context of marriage seemed almost too much to bear. Maybe they thought that Jesus would respond to them by lowering the standard set by God in creation, but instead, He pressed further to demonstrate the radical call of obedience to God and His kingdom. In essence, Jesus' response to His disciples in verses 11–12 teaches that if a person cannot abide by God's expectation for marriage, then it would actually be better for them to choose celibacy, that is, not to marry at all. If a person does not accept God's design for marriage—be that His design for marriage to be between one man and one woman or that marriage was to be a lifelong commitment where divorce is not considered an option unless one's spouse breaks the marriage covenant—then they should not get married.

To be sure, Jesus, along with Paul in 1 Corinthians 7, recognized that this teaching on willful celibacy for the sake of the kingdom was a teaching that not all could accept. To receive this teaching required the grace of God working in a person. Furthermore, neither Jesus' nor Paul's words should be construed as suggesting that celibacy was some higher calling or even a requirement for fruitful kingdom work. Instead, it was to demonstrate that God's ideal for marriage would not flex for those who found the standard too high.

God's standard for marriage, which Genesis 1–2 reveals and Jesus affirms in Matthew 19:1–12, won't be altered for those who refuse to conform to it. God's ideal for marriage is between one man and one woman for a lifetime. This ideal excludes the possibility of any other arrangement falling within God's boundaries for marriage. Marriage cannot be between a man and another man, nor between a woman and another woman. Furthermore, these categories of male and female are fixed at creation. A person cannot will themselves or change themselves in any meaningful way that can change how God has made them. Jesus unequivocally affirms and assumes this reality in His interactions with the Pharisees.

And if this calling for marriage was too high, then the only other acceptable option for those following Christ was celibacy. It would be better for a person to not marry at all than to violate God's ideal for marriage.

To some, this sounds harsh, but these are Jesus' words about marriage. Even He acknowledged that these teachings would be hard for some to receive. But if we understand Jesus' words as consistent with God's will (and we should!) and perceive Jesus to have God's glory and our good in mind, then we should not regard His words as harsh or unloving. He came that we might have life, "and have it to the full" (John 10:10), and this is not only referring to life in the future, but life right now. As Jesus prayed in John 17:3, "Now this is eternal life: that they know you, the only true God, and Jesus Christ, whom you have sent."

Life does not consist in the abundance of things, be those possessions or the freedom to engage in whatever sexual behaviors we desire. Life consists of knowing God in His manifold glory and living according to His Spirit instead of the desires of our flesh.

So, let's return to the statement "Jesus never spoke about homosexuality." Considering what Jesus consistently taught about sexual desires and marriage, it's hard to imagine that anyone could conclude that Jesus would have approved of homosexuality. Jesus not only warned us about the dangers of any sexual desire outside of the context of marriage, but He also conceived marriage as between one man and one woman for a lifetime. And this should come as no surprise from the Son of God, who came not to abolish God's law but to fulfill it. Thus, while we have no recording of Jesus speaking directly about homosexuality, He does, by implication, rule out the possibility that any sexual relationship outside of God's design for marriage is acceptable. Furthermore, He affirmed the authority of the Old Testament for revealing God's will for His creation, which explicitly addresses homosexuality. If someone attempts to build a case for the acceptability of homosexuality, they will have to look to someone other than Jesus. Jesus' views on marriage and sexuality are perfectly consistent with God's ideal for marriage, which He revealed in creation.

<hr />

We have considered God's good creation, what has gone wrong, and then delved into the issue of homosexuality in the Bible and whether or not Jesus really spoke on this topic. Next, we'll add to our biblical-theological framework as we discover Christ's loving mission: to seek and save the lost.

CHAPTER FIVE

Exploring the Biblical-Theological Framework Three

CHRIST: "To Seek and Save the Lost"

The older I get, the more sentimental I get. One of the things that gets me emotional is the clips of military parents being reunited with their kids. I love these videos! It might be a kid blindfolded in a martial arts class and being asked to defend themselves against a competitor only to take the blindfold off and see their father. Or it could be a mother who shows up unexpectedly at her daughter's pep rally. Or a brother who sends a video greeting to his sister at her graduation only to come up from behind the stage and greet her. It's like someone is cutting onions when I watch these videos!

I love these types of feel-good stories. We need more of them in our morbid news cycles. But they actually point to something bigger than the isolated events themselves. They point to our longing for bad or hard times to be resolved. For the crises to end and the celebrations to begin. The good news is that there is hope. While sin has left the world devastated, God did not turn His back on His creation. Instead, even before the foundation of the world was laid, God had a plan to redeem His creation and magnify His grace and mercy.

We see the first glimpse of this plan in Genesis 3:15 when God pronounces a curse on the serpent who had deceived the first humans. "And I will put enmity between you and the woman, and between your offspring and hers; he will crush your head, and you will strike his heel." Now, your first thought might be to read this passage as explaining why you are not very fond of snakes, but there is something bigger going on here that we need to be aware of. Some of the "oldest Jewish interpretations" of this passage take "the serpent as symbolic of Satan and look for a victory over him in the days of King Messiah."[1] New Testament authors pick up on this theme as well and apply this promise to Jesus and His subsequent followers (Rom. 16:20; Heb. 2:14). This led early church leaders like Justin Martyr and Irenaeus to dub Genesis 3:15 as the "protoevangelium," which is Latin for "first gospel."[2]

The idea here is that while the human author of Genesis might not have known exactly how God would fulfill this promise, God did and revealed, through a curse on the serpent, that one day, the deceiver would be destroyed through the work of the Son of God, Jesus Christ. Hence, Christian interpreters of Genesis 3:15 throughout the history of the church have taken this passage to be a glimpse of hope in an awful situation.

How would God deal with sin and evil? How would He crush the head of the deceiver and free His people from the destruction and devastation that ensued from sin's intrusion into creation? What was this gospel that was foreshadowed in the promise of Genesis 3:15?

We get a clearer picture of God's plan as we see the concept of sacrifice and atonement emerge in the Old Testament, especially in the context of the people of Israel.

Some wonder why it is important to read certain books in the Old Testament. Some of them can seem so strange to us. But if we want to understand what God was up to in the world and how He fulfilled His plan to deliver us from sin, we must take the Old Testament seriously. We cannot unhitch our understanding of God's plan

> For Adam and Eve to be covered, animals had to die. Thus, even at the beginning, we see God providing for His people through sacrifice.

for redeeming the world from the rich story and theology of the Old Testament. So, what does the Old Testament teach us about the concepts of sacrifice and atonement?

OUR NEED, GOD'S PROVISION

As I mentioned above, sacrifice and atonement emerge as we read the Old Testament. The first sacrifice is performed by God Himself in Genesis 3:21, where God provides clothing for Adam and Eve from the animal skins. While Genesis 3:7 tells us that Adam and Eve had made their own covering from fig leaves, they needed a covering that God would supply. Victor Hamilton noted this contrast between the fig leaves and the animal skins by stating, "The first is an attempt to cover oneself, the second is accepting a covering from another. The first is manmade and the second is God made. Adam and Eve are in need of a salvation that comes from without. God needs to do for them what they are unable to do for themselves."[3]

For Adam and Eve to be covered, animals had to die. Thus, even at the beginning, we see God providing for His people through sacrifice.[4] In Genesis 4, the idea of sacrifice comes up again. This time it is in the context of Cain and Abel, the offspring of Adam and Eve. Cain brings an offering of fruit, while Abel brings an offering from his flock. Genesis 4:4 describes Abel's offering as "fat portions from some of the firstborn of his flock." God accepts Abel's offering but rejects Cain's, which leads to Cain being filled with anger toward his brother and eventually murdering him. We are not told in Genesis 4 why God accepted Abel's offering but not Cain's offering, yet, in Hebrews 11:4, we learn that "by faith Abel brought God a better offering than Cain did." The fact that Genesis 4 mentions the "fat portions" and the "firstborn" probably indicates why God considered Abel's offering better.

As we keep reading through the Old Testament, all sorts of sacrifices appear repeatedly until we reach Exodus 12, where the Lord will deliver the people of Israel from Egyptian captivity. The final plague that the Lord will bring upon the Egyptians is the death of the firstborn in the land. Coupled with this plague is the establishment of the Passover with the Festival of the Unleavened Bread. As the Lord moved throughout the land, every home that followed Moses' instructions about Passover would be spared. An unblemished lamb would be killed and eaten while the blood of that lamb would be painted over the family's lintel and doorposts. When the Lord saw the blood, He would pass over the home.

For those who know the story, you are aware that the plague of the death of the firstborn quite literally passed over the homes of the Israelites who obey the Lord's command. After this plague, Moses led Israelites out of Egypt and into the wilderness for a journey into the promised land. As the people started their journey in the wilderness, the Lord gave more instruction through Moses to His people regarding how they should approach Him. Time and space would fail me to retell all of these details, but to summarize, it's during this time frame that the people learn about the tabernacle and the priesthood, who would oversee the sacrificial system to regulate their relationship with the Lord who had delivered them from Egypt. In time, the tabernacle, which represented the "ongoing presence" of the Lord among the people, would be supplanted by Solomon's temple, which was better suited for a people who had settled in the promised land.[5]

With each step forward in the story of Scripture, we witness God moving closer and closer to His people who had become estranged from Him due to their sin and rebellion until we reach the fulfillment of the promise made regarding the "Seed."[6] As Galatians 4:4–5 puts it, "But when the set time had fully come, God sent his Son, born of a woman, born under the law, to redeem those under the law, that we might receive adoption to sonship." Up until the coming of Christ, the Son of God, all the others who had been born of a woman failed to fulfill what God had promised in Genesis 3:15. Sin's curse hung over every man, woman, boy, and girl. No matter how many garments of fig leaves they had in their closets, they could not cover their own guilt, sin, and shame. God would have to do it for us, and that is exactly what He did in sending Christ Jesus into the world to save sinners like you and me.

This is where the light of the good news shines the brightest! But what exactly is it about this news that makes it so good? The apostle Paul gives us an answer in 1 Timothy 1:15. "Here is a trustworthy saying that deserves full acceptance: Christ Jesus came into the world to save sinners—of whom I am the worst." Let's break this "trustworthy saying" down a little more.

"CHRIST JESUS" . . .

Earlier in this chapter, we considered how some of the oldest Jewish interpretations of Genesis 3:15 believed that the promise would be fulfilled by the "Messiah King." We often encounter titles like "Messiah" or "Christ" and do not give them much thought, but this would not have been the case for the apostle Paul or other Jews in his day. For Paul to say "Christ Jesus" was another way of saying "Messiah King." This is also the way that other New Testament writers thought of Jesus.

Take, for instance, the opening of Matthew's gospel. Yes, the one with all the "begats" as King James phrases it, which tell us something about Jesus' family tree. Why would Matthew go to all the ancient trouble of compiling such a list at the beginning of his gospel? It's because Matthew was likely writing to a Jewish Christian audience to demonstrate, among many other things, "that Jesus is the promised Messiah, the Son of David, the Son of Man, Immanuel," which means "God with us."[7] Matthew wanted his readers to know that Jesus was the long-awaited Messiah, the offspring of David, who was promised in 2 Samuel 7:1–16. If you have ever visited a Christian church during the Advent season, you've likely heard readings and sung songs about this Old Testament promise that was fulfilled by the coming of Christ. That's what the Advent season is all about: a time of expectation and waiting when God would fulfill His promises to His people through the Christ, the Messiah, the King, who we know as Jesus.

It's at this point that I often see the most confusion about what it means to trust in Jesus and be saved from our sins. The vast majority of people who have some idea of their sinfulness are very receptive to the idea of a savior. And rightly so! I mean, who can blame them? And, just to be clear, Jesus is absolutely, as we will see below, the Savior of sinners. Yet, Jesus is not only our Savior, He is also our King or, as we often see Scripture refer to Him, our Lord. Most people like to view Jesus as their Savior, but not quite as many want Him as their King too. They want the benefits of Jesus' work on their behalf, but that's all they want from Him. They do not want to think of Jesus as having any real authority in their lives.

And I believe that is one of the main reasons many professing Christians are confused and questioning what the Bible teaches about sexuality.

If you have read or watched any recent material that argues for abandoning the sexual ethics that the Christian church has held for nearly two thousand years, you will likely find many people quoting the teachings of Jesus from the Gospels. These arguments are typically derived from teachings on "loving our neighbors." The

Some interpret loving our neighbors as "affirming" our neighbors.

command to "love our neighbors" is an important one. Jesus listed it right after stating that the greatest commandment is to love God with all our heart, soul, mind, and strength (see Mark 12:28–31). Obviously, loving our neighbors is a big deal. From here, the argument or the assumption is to interpret this idea of loving our neighbors as meaning something like "affirming" our neighbors.

We will see later why such an argument is wrong, but what I find interesting is that so little (if any) of this recent literature deals with Jesus' call to those who follow Him to "deny themselves and take up their cross" (Mark 8:34–38). The idea that following Jesus, truly trusting Him, would require me to give something up is foreign to so many people. People like seeing Jesus as a Savior but not a King. And when we fail to see Jesus as He has revealed Himself, the promised Son of Abraham, Son of David, the Christ, our whole vision of what it means to trust and follow Him gets skewed. So, we mustn't pass over quickly the significance of Jesus' title as the "Christ." If we do not embrace Him as He has revealed Himself, we will have no benefit from Him at all.

Thus, when we see Paul's brief description of the gospel in 1 Timothy 1:15, where he refers to Jesus as "Christ," we must recognize that he is drawing upon a rich history and tradition of expectation that God's chosen one, His King, would come into the world and deliver His people from the evil and brokenness that sin had brought into the world, which is exactly what we see in Paul's next statement.

"CAME INTO THE WORLD" . . .

The implication of the phrase "came into the world" is that something supernatural has occurred in the coming of Jesus, the Messiah King. Instead of dealing with our sin from afar, God took it personally, and in love "gave his one and only Son, that whoever believes in him shall not perish but have eternal life" (John 3:16). As Paul tells us in 1 Timothy 1:15, the Son of God came into the world as a man to deal with sin. Theologians call this event the incarnation, which speaks of the Son of God taking on flesh to become a human like us.

The author of Hebrews tells us why it was necessary for the Son of God to become a human like us. First, he tells us in Hebrews 2:14–15 that He shares in our humanity to break the power of the devil in our lives. Then, later in the book of Hebrews, we read, "We do not have a high priest who is unable to empathize with our weaknesses, but we have one who has been tempted in every way, just as we are—yet he did not sin" (Heb. 4:15).

John's gospel speaks of Jesus coming into the world in this way, "The Word became flesh and made his dwelling among us. We have seen his glory, the glory of the one and only Son, who came from the Father, full of grace and truth" (John 1:14). And, as we have already seen above, the apostle Paul describes this event in Galatians 4:4–5: "But when the set time had fully come, God sent his Son, born of a woman, born under the law, to redeem those under the law, that we might receive adoption to sonship."

"TO SAVE SINNERS"

Why did Christ Jesus come into the world? According to 1 Timothy 1:15, it was to save sinners. Sinners like Adam and Eve. Sinners like you and me. Sinners who, left to themselves, would be lost forever, condemned by our sinful rebellion to an eternal judgment under God's just wrath. Whatever other implications exist on account of Jesus' coming into the world (and there are many), He primarily came to save sinners from God's wrath (Rom. 5:6). The redemption of humanity from sin is the main reason Jesus came into the world. So, how did He do it? How did Jesus save sinners?

Scripture describes Jesus' work of saving sinners using various images. As we read the New Testament, we encounter terms like sacrifice, propitiation, reconciliation, and redemption employed to describe Jesus' saving work. The various images and terms bear witness to the magnitude of Jesus' work on behalf of sinners. No single word or image can fully contain all that Jesus did to save us, nor can I hope to expound all the riches contained in these words and images in a few short paragraphs. If, however, you forced me to give you one passage of Scripture that helpfully summarizes Jesus' saving work on our behalf, I would likely point you to Romans 3:21–26. Let's work through these verses together:

But now apart from the law the righteousness of God has been made known, to which the Law and the Prophets testify. This righteousness is given through faith in Jesus Christ to all who believe. There is no difference between Jew and Gentile, for all have sinned and fall short of the glory of God, and all are justified freely by his grace through the redemption that came by Christ Jesus. God presented Christ as a sacrifice of atonement, through the shedding of his blood—to be received by faith. He did this to demonstrate his righteousness, because in his forbearance he had left the sins committed beforehand unpunished—he did it to demonstrate his righteousness at the present time, so as to be just and the one who justifies those who have faith in Jesus.

First, we are told that God has made His righteousness known through Jesus Christ. In the life, death, burial, resurrection, and ascension of Jesus, we now have an even clearer picture of God's righteousness and our sinfulness. As the late John R. W. Stott put it, "Nothing reveals the gravity of sin like the cross. For ultimately what sent Christ there was neither the greed of Judas, nor the envy of the priests, nor the vacillating cowardice of Pilate, but our own greed, envy, cowardice and other sins, and Christ's resolve in love and mercy to bear their judgment and so put them away."[8] Nothing but the work of Jesus Christ, the Son of God, could save us.

God provided what God required through Christ, which is an atonement for our sins. But how do we receive the benefit of this atoning work?

But how? How did God save us? This is where the second point comes in. We are told that "God presented Christ as a sacrifice of atonement, through the shedding of his blood." William Tyndale likely coined the word "atonement" while translating the Bible in the sixteenth century. The idea was that this "sacrifice of atonement" brought back together a relationship that had been broken or severed due to an offense from one of the parties in the relationship. In humanity's case, sin was the offense that broke our relationship with God.

God's solution to this breach of relationship is "presenting Christ as a sacrifice of atonement, through the shedding of his blood," which reconciles sinners to Himself without forfeiting His righteousness in forgiving the sinner. The punishment that our sins deserve fell upon Christ, "the Lamb of God, who takes away the sin of the world" (John 1:29). In other words, God provided what God required through Christ, which is an atonement for our sins. But how do we receive the benefit of this atoning work? The passage tells us: this sacrifice of atonement is "to be received by faith."

This last phrase means that the benefits of Jesus' atoning death are received by us, not through our own works or efforts, but through trusting Jesus Christ "who had no sin to be sin for us, so that in him we might become the righteousness of God" (2 Cor. 5:21). By faith, we are united to Christ in His death and resurrection, which conquers the power of sin and death for us (1 Cor. 15:50–57). This gift of God is received by faith. It is not earned. It is not something that we work for. If we worked for it, it would not be a gift, but a wage owed to us. Instead, it is freely given to us, though it was of eternally great cost. And all who receive it by faith are declared righteous before God. Though we are all sinners by nature and by choice, through faith in Christ we can stand righteous, accepted before God, because of what He has done to save us. And unlike the sacrifices of the atonement in the Old Testament that had to be repeated with great regularity, Christ's sacrifice was "once for all" (Heb. 10:10).

BUT WAIT—THERE'S MORE!

At this point, you may be asking, "But what about the other things that have been broken by sin? Did Jesus do anything about those things?" He did! If all Jesus does is forgive our sins in this life and does not fix the brokenness that sin has caused in the world, if death itself is not vanquished that we may have eternal life in an eternal home with Him, can we really say that the gospel is good news? Christians have not always connected the significance of Christ's work to the whole creation, and that has led to some problems in the way that we think about salvation.

We must guard against losing our awe and wonder at the glory of God Himself who came to redeem us from sin. Yet, we must also understand that it was not just our sin that He came to redeem us from, but also the broken creation. In Romans 8:19–21, Paul tells us that even creation itself has been waiting for this day of redemption. He writes, "For the creation waits in eager expectation for the children of God to be revealed. For that creation was subjected to frustration, not by its own choice, but by the will of the one who subjected it, in hope that the creation itself will be liberated from its bondage to decay and brought into the freedom and glory of the children of God." What a thought! God has not abandoned us or the rest of His creation. Better things are coming for the children of God, and that's a truth you can bank on.

Let's conclude with some reflection.

1. How does my approach to sin and brokenness in the world magnify the person and work of Jesus Christ? In other words, considering what Christ has done, how does that impact how I think about sin and brokenness?

2. Does my perspective about sin and brokenness in the world reflect faith and confidence in the power of God in the gospel? Am I filled with despair when I observe the world, or hope because of God's mighty power through Christ?

I believe it is important for each of us to reflect on the gospel as we consider the problems we observe in the world. Observation of the world without meditation on the gospel of Christ will doubtlessly leave us full of anxiety and despair. Yet, if we remember what God has accomplished through Jesus, we do not need to fret. There is hope because of Jesus.

———

We have continued with our biblical-theological framework in discussing the joyous news that Christ has the answer to the world's being "not the way it's supposed to be," which is for any who will believe in Him. Next, we'll consider some of the practical applications of all this to issues we encounter as we determine to love our LGBTQ friends without compromising on biblical truth: a matter of identity; the wedding invitation; dinner around the table.

CHAPTER SIX

"Gay Christians"— Moral Identity and the Christian Life

W*ho are you?* What a question, right? There are all sorts of ways that people answer this question. It gets to the core of the idea of identity.

If someone asked me this question, I might be tempted to say, "I am a son, a brother, a husband, a father, a pastor, a professor, an author, a friend." Sounds like a typical social media bio, doesn't it? Had you asked me that question when I was younger, I would have confided that I was a future "shooting guard" in the NBA. God mercifully delivered me from this delusion once I attempted to play basketball as a freshman in high school.

So, my identity morphed into being a future golfer on the PGA Tour. Before Christ reached me, golf was my god. I dedicated almost every waking moment to learning the game. I got pretty good at it. I won a few local junior tournaments, but I only ever had interest from one Division 3 college that told me that I could come play but wouldn't receive a scholarship. When I asked about the community, I was told that the area was well known for its chicken farms. I told the coach I would be in touch, which was definitely a lie. Golf became a matter of recreation instead of vocation, and I set my sights on finding a job that paid a lot of money. Unfortunately, my lack of discipline in college outpaced my desire for riches.

During this time, though, God was working in my life through the preaching ministry of John Piper and the music of the late Keith Green. He was calling me into ministry, which, if I'm being honest, wasn't what I anticipated. In God's plan for me, I ended up getting a general studies degree and becoming an IT guy at a great local company with a Christian boss who allowed me to go to seminary while providing for my family. While in seminary, God's call on my life became clearer. He was calling me to be a pastor while getting further theological education, so I could play a role in training others for ministry. I never would have imagined during those days of dreaming about being a professional athlete that God would have different plans for me. In hindsight, though, I can say that I am grateful that His will, instead of my own, was done.

Each one of the identities that I have mentioned is or was true at some point in my life. But of all the identities that I have possessed in my life, the most essential and life-shaping identity that I have is this: "I am a Christian." I believe, as the Apostles' Creed puts it, that Jesus was born of the virgin Mary, suffered under Pontius Pilate, was dead, buried, rose again, and ascended into heaven, where He waits for the day when He will return and judge the world. As such, Jesus is both my Savior and my Lord. As my Savior, He has delivered me from the curse of sin by becoming a curse for me, in my place. He who knew no sin became sin so that *I might* become the righteousness of God in him (see 2 Cor. 5:21). In Christ, I have become a "new creation" (2 Cor. 5:17). When I was united to Jesus by faith, my identity fundamentally changed forever. All the other identities that I possess have now been brought under His lordship, His rule over me. I was bought with a price; therefore, everything that I do must aim to honor Him (1 Cor. 6:19–20). In Christ, I have lost self-ownership. I do not possess the right to answer the question "Who are you?" apart from reference to Christ's ownership of me. And if you are a Christian, I believe this is true of you as well.

The apostle Paul explains the significance of what has transpired for those who have put their trust in Jesus Christ. In Galatians 2:20, he writes, "I have been crucified with Christ. It is no longer I who live, but Christ who lives in me" (ESV). Through union with Christ by faith, we have died. Instead, Christ now lives in us. But what does that mean?

IDENTITY AND THE CHRISTIAN LIFE

In his book *Living in Union with Christ: Paul's Gospel and Christian Moral Identity*, Grant Macaskill argues that the problem with many conceptions of the Christian life is that "when we think about Christians as moral agents who act within the church and the world in an ethically good way, we conceive of their agency in terms that are not properly determined by who Jesus is and how he is present in them."[1] The problem, as Macaskill understands it, is that such a conception of moral agency excludes Christ from being "personally involved in the *believer's* obedience." The result is a "self-centered" approach to "moral activity or growth" that while relying upon the Spirit is still "something *we* do."[2] In other words, instead of placing our union with Christ in the background, it should be in the foreground. When we answer the question "Who are you?" our response should reflect the centrality of Christ in us.

Macaskill goes on to contend that

> Paul's account of the Christian life involves a rejection of the idea that our natural selves can ever be improved or repaired in their own right. . . . Their only prospect for salvation lies in their being inhabited by another self, a better self who can act in them to bring about real goodness. Hence, Paul's personal hope is expressed in his statement "It is no longer I who live, but Christ who lives in me" (Gal. 2:20).[3]

Any account of the Christian moral life, any program of discipleship, that does not begin and resolve with Paul's words, "I no longer live, but Christ lives in me," is deficient and will eventually turn into a form of idolatry.

Obviously, Galatians 2:20 plays a crucial role in Macaskill's argument about identity, and I believe it is significant for us to consider. What Christ has done for us is not just a matter of forgiving our sins, but also a matter of granting us a new identity in Him. And this new identity comes with moral implications that Christ Himself is at work to accomplish His will in us.

Macaskill continues, "Any account of the Christian moral life, any program of discipleship, that does not begin and resolve with Paul's words, 'I no longer live, but Christ lives in me,' is deficient and will eventually turn into a form of idolatry."[4]

In other words, when we exclude Christ from our understanding of who we are, things will not go well. Our desires will turn away from

God to other sources of identity and idolatry, which essentially means we will look to other "gods" instead of our Creator God for instruction on how to live and find meaning in this world. This is precisely what I did at different stages of my life and am still tempted to do.

Consider the temptation a pastor faces to find their identity, the answer to their "who am I," in their vocation. Suppose a pastor's sense of worth or significance is based on how their church is perceived to be doing compared to other churches. In that case, they will ride a roller coaster of excitement and disappointment every week. One week, the offering is strong, all the volunteers show up on time, and people tell him how great the sermon was as they dismiss the service. The next week, the offering doesn't cover the expenses, multiple volunteers cancel, and the only thing he hears as people leave is that it was too hot in the sanctuary. A success, blessed and highly favored by the Lord one week. A failure, full of doubt and worry that the Lord has abandoned his ministry altogether the next.

Do you see how dangerous it is to find our sense of identity outside of Christ? What we need as the bedrock of our identity is the immovable foundation of Christ Jesus as our Lord and Savior. This reality must not only shape but sometimes, when necessary, displace other identities that rival the transformative power of Christ's presence in us. So, what does the transformative power of Christ's presence in us mean?

BEING CONFORMED TO HIS IMAGE

Here is where I believe that what we have seen from Grant Macaskill's *Living in Union with Christ* makes a huge difference in our perspective on personal identity. I love how Macaskill frames this idea. He writes that the apostle "is not becoming a better version of Paul; he is becoming Paul-in-Christ. He is metamorphosing into the likeness of Jesus."[5] This idea of "metamorphosing" is grounded in the language of Romans 8:29 and 12:2, which reminds us that it's the image of Christ to which we're to become conformed, not the pattern of the world. Our aim is not to become splendid highly moral versions of ourselves, but that we exhibit His moral identity. Thinking about our identity in this order prioritizes not only who Christ is and what He has done, but also considers what He is actively doing through the Holy Spirit now to make us like Himself. Understood in this way, Christ is not simply an instrument to form us but rather the substance of our identity. It is no longer "I" who live, but Christ who lives in me.

The implication of Christ's living in us is that all other identities that we may bear must now be subjected to, tested by, and transformed in relationship to the One who dwells in us by the Holy Spirit.

If this is the case, then what is the Holy Spirit's role? We do not rely on the Spirit to help us fulfill a potential to be a better "I," but to mature us in our identity as conforming to the Son. Because we are sinners, we are not able to create better versions of ourselves on our own but need someone else: the Spirit *of* the Son (Gal. 4:6). In other words, our greatest need cannot be solved by us. It must come from Christ working through the Spirit. All of us are desperately corrupted by sin and need more than improvement. We need Christ to take up residence in us, which leads to us taking on a new identity.

The implication of Christ's living in us is that all other identities that we may bear must now be subjected to, tested by, and transformed in relationship to the One who dwells in us by the Holy Spirit. Where these other identities conform to the will of the One who dwells in us, that may be retained. We see this in how Paul talks about his own apostleship. Even though he regards himself as having died with Christ, his identity as an apostle is consistent with "Christ-in-Paul." However, when he perceives there to be an identity crisis within himself, where there is a temptation to elevate or take pride in one of his secondary identities, Paul sees the need to put that identity to death. Notice the radical way that Paul speaks of this in Philippians 3:3–11:

> For it is we who are the circumcision, we who serve God by his Spirit, who boast in Christ Jesus, and who put no confidence in the flesh—though I myself have reasons for such confidence.
>
> If someone else thinks they have reasons to put confidence in the flesh, I have more: circumcised on the eighth day, of the people of Israel, of the tribe of Benjamin, a Hebrew of Hebrews; in regard to the law, a Pharisee; as for zeal, persecuting the church; as for righteousness based on the law, faultless.
>
> But whatever were gains to me I now consider loss for the sake of Christ. What is more, I consider everything a loss because of the surpassing worth of knowing Christ Jesus my Lord, for whose sake I have lost all things. I consider them garbage, that I may gain Christ and be found in him, not having a righteousness of my own that comes from the law, but that which is through faith in Christ—the righteousness that comes from God on the basis of faith. I want to know Christ—yes, to know the power of his resurrection and participation in his sufferings, becoming like him in his death, and so, somehow, attaining to the resurrection from the dead.

Was it a sin for Paul to acknowledge that he was "a Hebrew of Hebrews"? Of course not. It was part of his story and God's story.

Yet this identity, as true as it may have been, was not the primary, controlling identity that Paul possessed or strove to attain. In fact, in comparison to the identity he possessed in Christ, Paul regarded all other identities as loss. Their worth could not compare to the worth of knowing and being known by Christ as a participant in His death and resurrection.

The question for us is whether Christians should think in such terms about their identity. Should this struggle with same-sex attraction be considered part of who they are?

Taking our lead from Scripture, we need to recognize the centrality of our identity in Christ. Whenever we are tempted to let all the other identities that we possess creep into the center and become the control descriptor of who we are and how we feel, we must resist and return to what we have been taught. It is no longer I who live, but Christ who lives in me. So, what bearing does this teaching have on the relatively recent phenomenon of professing Christians describing themselves as "gay"?

"GAY CHRISTIAN"

Mostly, when I have encountered professing Christians using the word "gay" as a description, it typically means something like "I am a Christian who experiences same-sex attraction." In other words, "gay" is viewed as part of their identity, which is related to what we have seen described early in chapter 3 regarding the APA's definition of sexual orientation. Often there's a distinction being made between orientation and behavior. Many Christians who describe themselves as gay would affirm that God's Word clearly prohibits same-sex behavior. The debate, then, is not so much about behavior but rather how to make sense of the desires that these Christians wrestle with as they seek to live faithfully to Christ.

The question for us is whether Christians should think in such terms about their identity. Should this struggle with same-sex attraction be considered part of who they are? In order to answer this question, we need to attempt to answer two other questions first: "Can and should our identity in Christ receive a modifier?" and "Is same-sex attraction sinful?"

A MODIFIED IDENTITY?

At first glance, our default response to the first question above might be, "Of course not. Why would our identity in Christ need any modification?" This is true. Yet by asking, we're not somehow suggesting our identity in Christ might have a modifier. Rather, we are acknowledging that—though our identity in Christ is central—it does not mean that all other identity markers lose any descriptive or theological benefit.

Consider how Revelation 5 speaks of people from every "tribe and language and people and nation" surrounding the throne in heaven with praise to the Lamb who was slain. I love the glory of this scene in heaven! Heaven is a place full of ethnic diversity, which is clear from the language that John uses to describe it. Every "tribe and language and people and nation" has representatives there, praising the worthiness of Jesus, the Lamb of God! There is no hint in this passage that these real distinctions that exist among the people of the earth get erased. There are no gated communities or urban blight in this place. No, just the glory of God among peoples redeemed by the blood of Jesus. I say all this to temper our temptation to say that there is no biblical basis for acknowledging real though secondary differences among those who bear that same identity together in Christ. But what about other real differences?

Well, one that seems clear is that there are real differences between men and women. Not only does the creation account point to this reality, but also the different roles and responsibilities we can observe in households, churches, and the world. While men and women both share in the divine image of God and are worthy of respect, love, and value, they are also different by God's design. Consider the different roles of husbands and wives or fathers and mothers in the household codes of the New Testament.

It was no contradiction for Paul to be both an apostle and a tentmaker so long as Christ remained central to his identity.

Another area of real difference that we have already alluded to in the heavenly scene from Revelation 5 is that of nationality or place of origin. Again, there is nothing inherently wrong with acknowledging these distinctions. We see Scripture making these distinctions regularly. Just think of how Luke, a Greek physician turned traveling missionary, describes issues between the Hebraic and Hellenistic widows in Acts 6.

There is legitimacy in seeing real differences between people who bear the same identity in Christ. Consider the different vocations mentioned in the Bible. Paul, for one, while an apostle of Jesus Christ, was also a tentmaker. It was no contradiction for Paul to be both an apostle and a tentmaker so long as Christ remained central to his identity. Or what about the Christians who still maintained a role in the Roman Empire after their conversion? What about the amanuensis that Paul mentions in his letters?

Obviously, this is not an exhaustive consideration of the various identities that are mentioned in Scripture, but they do give us a glimpse into how to navigate finding our fundamental identity in Christ while serving in the other roles that God has assigned us in this life. With that said, however, I want us to note something about these identities that we have considered. None of these identities appear to conflict with Christ's work by the Holy Spirit to be formed in us. Nothing about being a man or a woman, a husband or a wife, a tentmaker or a professional scribe conflicts with being conformed to the image of God in Christ. And I think this is an important thing to note as we make these observations about identity. We should be careful with how we identify ourselves, considering our identity in Christ. As a principle, if Christ would not have used the language that we have chosen as a description, we should not use it either.

If we are not careful here, we might very well find ourselves using a description of ourselves that works against the work that God is doing in us. For instance, I think that most of you would find it odd if someone described themselves as a "Christian atheist." Something about that self-description would make you want to say, "There is a competing vision here. This seems contrary to what God is working in us." I believe that inclination is right, which leads us to the next question: Is same-sex attraction sinful?

IS SAME-SEX ATTRACTION SINFUL?

Even posing this question causes discomfort. If, as many have argued, "same-sex attraction" is innate, that is, involuntary for some people, how could a person be culpable for something that appears to be outside of their control? I mean, who would blame a child with Tourette's Syndrome for moving or making sounds in a classroom? Doesn't the involuntary nature of the action remove the culpability of the person experiencing it? If the behavior does not spring from our will, how could we be held accountable for it?

This question has certainly provoked some heated debates within the evangelical church, and I doubt that my answer will please everyone. I realize there are different opinions on this question. Furthermore, I'm not saying you have to agree with me to be a Christian. I'm simply going to give my best attempt to answer the question as I understand it.

So, first, I think it is important for us to go back to the definition of sin that we saw earlier in the book. Sin was defined as "whatever is opposed to God's will, as that will reflects God's holy character and as that will is expressed by God's commands."[6] Assuming this definition, then, we can ask, "Is same-sex attraction opposed to God's will?" Given what we have already seen regarding God's very good ideal for sex in creation and His instructions about sex in His Word, I believe that the answer to this question is "Yes. Same-sex attraction is opposed to God's will." Same-sex sexual attraction and desire are contrary to God's will for His creation.

But how does this answer consider those desires and attractions that appear to be involuntary for some people? You might conclude that those who willfully embrace and celebrate their same-sex attraction are sinning, but what about those who hate these desires yet experience them nonetheless? Isn't the implication of my answer that same-sex attracted people are hopelessly and irredeemably trapped with a sinful desire they cannot escape?

To answer these questions, we must consider a few other things about sin and our relationship to it. The first thing that we need to see is that we inherited our disposition toward sin from the first man, Adam. Romans 5:12–14 teaches us this, stating, "Therefore, just as sin entered the world through one man, and death through sin, and in this way death came to all people, because all sinned—To be sure, sin was in the world before the law was given, but sin is not charged against anyone's account where there is no law. Nevertheless, death reigned from the time of Adam to the time of Moses, even over those who did not sin by breaking a command, as did Adam, who is a pattern of the one to come."

Another key passage that speaks of the result of Adam's sin for all humanity comes from 1 Corinthians 15:22, which says, "For as in Adam all die, so in Christ all will be made alive." To be brief, in these two passages, Paul compares Adam and Christ. In and through Adam, sin and death spread to all people. As descendants of Adam, we inherit a sinful nature and suffer the consequences of sin, even before we are aware of sin. Every aspect of our lives is tainted by our sinful nature, which we did not ask for or willfully choose. Another way to state this would be to say that Adam was the representative of all humanity. We bear a solidarity with Adam as his descendants. And when he rebelled against God, the punishment for his sin was not only experienced by him but all creation.

Now, at first glance, this appears to be wildly unfair, especially to those of us who have been raised in the individualistic cultures of the West. Why would I be held accountable for someone else's sin? This just doesn't seem right. But I would caution us from allowing our Western values to shape our understanding of fairness. When God reveals how He intends to relate to us, He does not have to ask us for permission. The Creator does not have to consult His creation, nor can what He has created respond to Him and protest, "Why have you created me this way?" We must remember the important distinction between the Creator and the creation.

Now, if you think that being represented by Adam is unfair, please hold your evaluations until the end of the story. Why? Because God has provided another representative for humanity! This is the point that Paul is driving at in Romans and 1 Corinthians. While Adam has failed, God's new representative did not fail. Who is this representative? Christ Himself! For while we were destined for death and condemnation due to Adam's sin and our own, God sent His Son into the world, unstained by sin, to live in perfect obedience to His will and destroy death through His own death and resurrection. Thus, in Christ, not only is perfect righteousness earned through His obedience to all of God's will, but the penalty of death that hangs over all sinners is paid in full through His atoning sacrifice. Therefore, all who are united to Christ by faith now enjoy the benefits He earned for us as our representative.

If being represented by Adam seemed unfair, how would we ever accept Christ's representation for us? In Christ, the penalty has been paid for us! In Christ, the righteous life that we were incapable of living due to our sinful nature and sinful action has been lived for us! The curse that fell on all creation because of Adam's rebellion has, is, and will be ultimately removed for all who are found to be in Christ.

Why have I gone to the trouble of explaining this theological component of our struggle with sin? It's because we need to have some understanding of our nature as sinners if we are going to answer a question about the sinfulness of our desires, even those that seem involuntary. When assessing the morality of our desires, the question is not ultimately about whether the desires were voluntary or involuntary, but rather, how those desires reflect God's will. This is the fundamental question, not "Do I or do I not want to do this or that?"

Before we ever get to the question of our willingness to do something, we must remember that before our union with Christ, all our desires were downstream from our death in Adam. Furthermore, even once we have been united with Christ by faith, we still carry around this "body that is subject to death" (Rom. 7:24). Paul goes on to talk about this struggle between the flesh and the Spirit in Romans 8:10–11, where he writes, "But if Christ is in you, then even though your body is subject to death because of sin, the Spirit gives life because of righteousness. And if the Spirit of him who raised Jesus from the dead is living within you, he who raised Christ from the dead will also give life to your mortal bodies because of his Spirit who lives in you."

So, there is a sense in which we carry around two natures in us. These two natures are constantly competing for our allegiance. One nature is life in the Spirit, which Paul says brings about righteousness in us. When we live in the life of the Spirit, we are mindful of our need to "put to death the misdeeds" (Rom. 8:13) of the body/flesh, which is the second nature that we carry around in us. The nature of life in the body/flesh is the life of sin and rebellion against God, which we inherited from Adam. By the indwelling presence and power of the Holy Spirit, the life of the body/flesh that we were once enslaved to can now be put to death. In fact, as Paul would say, it must be "put to death" (v. 13). Before we were united to Christ, we were only aware of the life of the body/flesh (Rom. 7:5). But now, in Christ, we not only possess and are called to live in the life of the Spirit, but we have an awareness of the life of the body/flesh that must be resisted and put to death on a daily basis. It is how we live until the fullness of our redemption in Christ is realized,

We do not minimize or trivialize the severity and intensity of the struggle against the desires of our sinful nature.

giving us a helpful category for understanding this ongoing tension between the two natures we carry around with us. Here in Romans 7 and 8, Paul sets before us two ways of living: one according to our sin nature, the other according to our new nature in Christ by the Spirit.

What this means for our question of whether "same-sex attraction is sinful" is that we can affirm that same-sex attraction is sinful. It is contrary to God's will for us. It is a desire that arises from our sin nature. Yet, it is also possible for us to affirm that one's struggle with same-sex attraction is not definitive for understanding one's new life in Christ. Yes, the desires may persist, just as we know that many other sinful desires (e.g., anger, jealousy, gluttony) persist until the day of our full redemption in Christ. But that does not mean that we should be apathetic to such desires or that we should believe that there is no hope for escape from these desires. That is emphatically not what Paul is teaching us in these verses. Instead, because of the life of the Spirit living within us, we have the obligation and power to resist the desires of our sinful nature. We were incapable of doing this before our union with Christ. For, as Paul tells us in Romans 8:11, God is at work in us by His Spirit to produce life within us, which is another way of saying that He is working to conform us now in the present with the fullness of life that we will experience totally with the resurrection of our bodies. For any believer to accept the desires of their sinful nature as some destiny or will of God for their lives is to functionally deny the presence and power of the Holy Spirit who is at work within us to produce life that accords with God's will.

This, of course, is not to minimize or trivialize the severity and intensity of the struggle against the desires of our sinful nature. Any professing Christian who would say to a fellow brother or sister in Christ who struggles with same-sex attraction, "Oh, just get over it and move on," demonstrates a naïveté about the war being waged (Rom. 7:22–25) between the flesh and the Spirit within us. War is hard, and as loving brothers and sisters in Christ, we ought to lock arms with one another in this war against our sinful nature together. When we gather with one another, wars are raging within all of us. We need to demonstrate humility, love, patience, prayerfulness, compassion, and sympathy to our fellow soldiers in this war against our sinful natures, ceaselessly reminding each other that there is a day coming when the war will cease when we see Him face to face. Until that day, though, we must fight in the strength that He provides, not against each other, but against the one who rages against all of us (Eph. 6:10–20).

SHOULD CHRISTIANS DESCRIBE THEMSELVES AS "GAY" OR "SAME-SEX ATTRACTED"?

This question brings us back to the whole question about identity. One of the most helpful things I have read on this topic comes from Rachel Gilson. In her book *Born Again This Way*, she makes an important differentiation between the type of markers that I mentioned earlier (gender, vocation, etc.) and those that are related to our fallen nature as a sinner. Gilson makes the point that while her gender (female) is not tied to her fallen nature, her same-sex attractions are. She writes,

> They are true in the sense that they exist. They are important, especially because the culture presses us to treat them as safe and good while Scripture presses us to soberly flee temptation of all kinds. They must be denied, in the sense that we must say no to their demands for same-gender sex and romance. But they need

not be denied in the sense of going unacknowledged. We can't make war with an opponent while stopping our eyes and ears to their whereabouts.[7]

Gilson is right about the importance of naming and acknowledging those aspects of our lived experience that are due to our fallen nature. Furthermore, I deeply appreciate the imagery she employs regarding the spiritual warfare that all Christians are engaged in. If people mean what Gilson means when they say that they are "same-sex attracted," then I can almost get onboard, but I do have one point of hesitation.

The problem is not with what Gilson states, but rather with a possible misunderstanding that others could take from it. While I fully appreciate what Gilson and others have written on the importance of naming one's struggle with same-sex attraction, I do wonder about the long-term benefits of such a designation. The point that Gilson makes about the need to acknowledge the struggle against same-sex attraction makes sense. How can you fight an enemy that you do not acknowledge? This is a good point. My concern lies in allowing such a struggle to creep into such a place of prominence in the believer's life that they inadvertently make the struggle against their same-sex attraction the litmus test of their sanctification. Let me see if I can illustrate the danger I perceive here.

Back in college, I met regularly with other Christian men in an accountability group. We would get together, enjoy some Taco Bell, open our Bibles, and then ask each other, "How are you doing?" It was rare for us to gather for one of these meetings and someone not to mention that they were struggling with lust, which was often manifesting in a relationship or in pornography use. Unfortunately, we often viewed our struggle against our flesh to be so narrow that if, in the prior week, we had experienced victory over lust, we would conclude that we were "doing well."

I am not suggesting that there was anything wrong with these honest accountability meetings. It was right to acknowledge our struggles. It was right and good for us to confess our sins and remind each other of the assurance of pardon we possessed in Christ. But the struggle against lust kind of became the essence of our struggle against the flesh, which I feel left our group open to an inflated view of our spiritual progress at times. I don't recall anyone ever bringing up their struggle against slothfulness or gluttony in those meetings. Yet, there we were, eating crazy amounts of food chased by copious amounts of Mountain Dew, staying up to ridiculous hours in the night, and sleeping till noon the next day. But hey, as long as we were not doing anything particularly immoral with our girlfriends or looking at porn on the computer, we were "doing well," right?

We need to be careful in our acknowledgment of our particular struggles with sexual immorality not to give those struggles such a controlling place in the narrative of our spiritual growth that they become the sole or primary test of our conformity to Christ. Our enemy, the devil, is just as pleased to destroy us with sloth and gluttony as he is to destroy us with desires for sexual immorality. It really makes no difference to him. Whatever can be used to take our eyes off Christ, he's fine with it.

So, while I agree with Gilson about the need to name and acknowledge our particular struggles against sin, I also want to caution us from declaring those struggles to be unchangeable to the point that they shape our understanding of what it means to be conformed to Christ. It seems her point is about acknowledging in order to go to war with those desires that we experience, which are contrary to God's will for us. To that, I say, "Amen!" I just also want us all to be clear that if we woke up one day and experienced complete victory over a particular sin, that victory should be regarded as a battle victory, not a war victory. The battle victories are steps along the way to the war victory, which Christ has secured for His people. Another way of stating this would be to say that the goal of our conformity to Christ is not merely the alleviation of same-sex attraction, but rather, the full removal of all sinful desires that do not accord with God's will.

WHAT IF THE SAME-SEX ATTRACTIONS NEVER GO AWAY?

In one sense, we could answer this question by saying, "All sinful desires will eventually go away when we will be completely conformed to the image of Christ." I bet most people asking this question already knew that answer, but they are concerned mainly with their life before Christ's return. The question is more likely, "Will I always have to struggle with these attractions? Will I ever experience a full victory over these sinful impulses in this life? And if I don't, what does that mean for me?"

These are hard questions to answer. In fact, I would venture to say they are impossible to answer because to answer them would require access to the mind of God. I simply don't know. Is it possible that these same-sex attractions could disappear one day in this life? Absolutely. Is it *certain* that they will disappear in this life? I cannot say that it is. What I do know is that we will and must struggle and fight against sin until the day we die or Christ returns.

When this body of flesh, with all of its misdeeds and desires, is finally laid to rest in the ground or transformed at the appearing of Christ, then, and only then, will our fight against sin be over. So, it's entirely possible that you or someone you know may struggle and fight against same-sex attraction for the rest of their lives on this earth. This is true of every Christian that has ever lived, regardless of the sins that they are waging war against. But thanks be to God that there is a day of victory of the flesh coming for all who are in Christ!

If you're someone who struggled with same-sex attraction, this is no mere intellectual question. It's a desperate one. You may ask, "But why? Why wouldn't God just free me totally, right now, from this struggle?" This is such a deep question.

In my own wrestling with sins that seem to be a daily struggle for me, I have found great comfort in the wisdom and sovereignty of God over my life. How does the wisdom and sovereignty of God over my life comfort me in the daily struggle with sins? Let me share something that revolutionized my way of thinking about the struggle.

It comes from John Piper's foreword to John Owen's book *Overcoming Sin and Temptation*. Piper noted some of the nuggets of truth that lie within Owen's book. I'll never forget reading the paragraph and calling my brother. It was a perspective that I had never considered, but I hope it is beneficial to you, just as it was for me. Owen wrote, "God says, 'Here is one, if he could be rid of this lust I should never hear of him more; let him wrestle with this, or he is lost.'" Piper goes on to comment on Owen's point here, "Astonishing! God ordains to leave a lust with me till I become the

For those who struggle with same-sex attraction daily, who wonder why God has not answered your prayers for the desires to be removed, it may be because God loves you and knows you well enough to know what victories you can and can't handle right now.

sort of warrior who will still seek his aid when this victory is won.

God knows when we can bear the triumphs of his grace."[8]

Did you catch that? Owen essentially answered our question by saying that sometimes God allows us to keep struggling with a particular sin (his term, lust) because He knows that if we were freed from the struggle, we would move on with our life in our own strength with no regard for our daily need for Him. That's really deep, but it's also very comforting. It is comforting to know that God is not only working in the lives of believers to conform them to Christ, but He is even working in our struggles against sin. For me, it's meant that maybe the reason why I have not seen the victory over my sin of worry yet is because God knows that I am not yet mature enough to handle "the triumphs of his grace" over it. My struggle drives me to my knees daily. It causes me to plead with God for His mercy and grace, asking Him to increase my faith so that I might put my worry to death by the power of the Holy Spirit. And by allowing me to continue to struggle with the sin of worry, God is forming my identity in Christ in the fight of faith. He is showing me just how dependent I am on Him for everything.

For those who struggle with same-sex attraction daily, who wonder why God has not answered your prayers for the desires to be removed, it may be because God loves you and knows you well enough to know what victories you can and can't handle right now. As Owen noted, maybe God knows that if I were completely freed from my struggle with worry or you were completely freed from your struggle with same-sex attraction, we would not look to Him as we do now. We might carry on with our lives in our own strength, thinking that because we have had a victory over these particular sins, now we do not need Him. "God knows when we can bear the triumphs of his grace."

In God's wisdom and sovereignty, He knows what's best for shaping our identity in greater conformity to Christ. While all sorts of struggles with sin will persist until the day when we are completely free, we can trust that God is at work by His Spirit to make us more like Jesus. There is peace here. May the Lord give us eyes to see it, ears to hear it, and the faith to receive it, as Christ, the hope of glory, is formed in us.

CHAPTER SEVEN

"Will We See You at the Wedding?"— Gay Marriage

I don't exactly love weddings. Don't get me wrong, I enjoy celebrating with friends and family. But as a pastor, I am sometimes asked to officiate weddings, and I have a nagging fear that I will ruin someone else's special day.

Consider what happened to me at a recent wedding. It was an outdoor ceremony, and as I was speaking to the bride and groom, a small bug flew into my mouth. Internally, I panicked. In between each word that I spoke, I could feel the bug moving. What should I do? Should I stop speaking and stick my fingers in my mouth? Do I turn my head and spit? Well, I'm a little proud and embarrassed to say it, but I decided to chew the bug up in between words and then swallow it. No one noticed that this happened. The special day was preserved. And as a bonus, I got a mid-ceremony snack. But maybe now you understand why I would much rather attend than officiate because then the pressure would be off me to ensure everything went off without a hitch.

Weddings are special times. There is laughter, great food, good music, and much fellowship. We reunite with old friends and family. We give gifts. We dress up. We decorate the getaway car. And we wish the bride and groom a happily ever after. No wonder people are kind enough to invite us to these special gatherings. They want us to be with them and celebrate. So, we "save the date," RSVP, travel if necessary, and attend to show our support.

But what are Christians to do when the wedding that they have been invited to does not align with what God's Word teaches about marriage? For instance, what should a Christian do if they are invited to a gay wedding? How do we navigate such a potentially divisive situation? And, most importantly, how do we do this while showing love without compromising the truth?

WEDDINGS IN OUR CHRISTIAN CONTEXT

For the most part, weddings are times of celebration. One of the first events we see Jesus attend is a wedding in Cana. In John 2:1–12, Jesus performs His first miracle at this celebration, turning water into wine. I can still remember the first time I taught on this miracle in a rather conservative church. It was during a Wednesday night prayer meeting, which typically involved some feedback. At the end of the teaching session, I asked if there were any questions or comments. A woman raised her hand to object. She told me that the reason that Jesus did this was not because He approved of the wine but because the water was not safe to drink. I should have been prepared for such a comment. I mean, I was talking about wine to a congregation of likely teetotalers! But alas, I just didn't think that anyone would see a problem with it. I could have pointed out that just a few chapters later in the gospel of John, Jesus asks a Samaritan woman for a drink of water from the well, which presumably would have been drinkable. Instead I said, "Well, if Jesus had the power to turn water into wine, then surely He could have turned dirty water into drinkable water." I don't think she was entirely happy with my answer. But maybe we were both focused on the wrong thing. In Bible times, wine was associated with joy. When the wine ran out, the joy was gone. And Jesus miraculously enabled the party to continue. Jesus wasn't afraid of a celebration.

But Jesus wasn't just a wedding attender, He also participates in one as well—a divine, cosmic one. In Revelation 19:6–9, we read, "Then I heard what sounded like a great multitude, like the roar of rushing waters and like loud peals of thunder, shouting: 'Hallelujah! For our Lord God Almighty reigns. Let us rejoice and be glad and give him glory! For the wedding of the Lamb has come, and his bride has made herself ready. Fine linen, bright and clean, was given her to wear.' (Fine linen stands for the righteous acts of God's holy people.) Then the angel said to me, 'Write this: Blessed are those who are invited to the wedding supper of the Lamb!' And he added, 'These are the true words of God.'"

In the midst of the planning, we need to pay careful attention to the importance of the words spoken by the minister and the vows made between husband and wife.

By invoking the imagery of a wedding, we see the reward that has been promised to those who hold fast to Christ pictured as a wedding celebration.

Another way of thinking about this is to see that marriage from beginning to end is God's idea. It is an important idea for understanding God's design not only for humanity but also for the end goal of our redemption in Christ. Jesus will receive His bride, the church. And, while there is no need to extrapolate undue parallels between the marriage supper of the Lamb and His bride and our earthly marriages, it is also not without warrant to see that our marriages point to an even greater reality. This was Paul's point in Ephesians 5:32. Given the great reality that our earthly marriages point to, we must realize that we are not free to make marriages or our weddings primarily about us.

In addition to seeing weddings as celebrations, we should also see them as ceremonies. There is a beauty and order to a wedding ceremony. We wear special clothes and decorate in extravagant ways. We serve good food and drinks. We aim to cultivate a memorable experience both for the wedding party and all the guests. In the midst of the planning that goes into these sacred ceremonies, we sometimes need to pay careful attention to the importance of the words spoken by the minister and the vows made between husband and wife. These vows are not inconsequential. They are made before God and a host of other witnesses. They carry both spiritual and legal weight. To make a vow before God and others is to agree to something far more important than a home mortgage or a car payment.

It seems the practice of addressing those attending a wedding and asking, "If anyone can show just cause why this couple cannot lawfully be joined together in holy matrimony, let them speak now or forever hold their peace," was formalized in the Book of Common Prayer in 1549. It was part of the church's role in solemnizing a marriage. As the story goes, news traveled slowly in the sixteenth century, and record-keeping was not the highest priority. This meant that churches would typically announce a wedding a few weeks in advance of the actual date to give people adequate time to voice any questions they had about the marriage's legality. I know that this might seem a little weird in today's world, but this practice points to the community's witness in the marriage ceremony. When we attend a wedding, we are not just simply celebrating; we are also lending our endorsement, our approval to the marriage itself. So, how do these truths help us answer our question about attending a same-sex wedding?

IN THE PRESENCE OF THESE WITNESSES

I believe Christians ought to refrain from attending any wedding that does not conform to God's design for marriage. This would apply not only to same-sex weddings, which cannot actually be marriages, but also other weddings that celebrate a union that undermines the one-flesh union between a husband and a wife. Same-sex weddings and the subsequent marriages that they supposedly solemnize are not weddings or marriages in God's eyes. A Christian must conform to God's intent for marriage—after all, it was His idea, not ours— rather than to what the culture or state declares is a marriage. We are not free to redefine marriage, nor are we free to celebrate that which God Himself does not recognize. But I would go even a step further.

Not only should Christians not lend their support to a same-sex wedding, but they should not support any wedding that violates God's design for marriage. What am I talking about here? I'm saying that before we ever got to the question of same-sex weddings, some Christians played fast and loose with God's design for marriage by tolerating marriages that did not please God.

Take, for instance, the case of a man and a woman who get married to each other after one or both have been divorced for unbib- lical reasons. Let's say that they met while married to their former spouse and committed adultery. Biblically speaking, while their new marriage is technically recognized as a marriage, it is also viewed as having been conceived in adultery. Such a marriage is also contrary to God's design for marriage. Except in cases where a spouse dies or the marriage covenant was broken through sexual immorality or abandonment (which I believe would include abuse), the offending or guilty spouse should not remarry. If, however, the guilty spouse remarries, the Bible teaches that they have committed adultery. As such, a Christian should not endorse or support such a marriage through their attendance at the wedding. We might not always have these details, but when we do, we should be mindful of what we are saying to the world by supporting a marriage that God Himself would not support.

That might seem harsh to you, even judgmental. I know. But again, marriage is God's idea, not ours; therefore, we should be discerning in what we support. Part of the reason that we are even having the conversation about same-sex marriage in our society is because we have consistently devalued marriage through our toleration of no-fault divorce and easy remarriage. I am under no delusion that everyone will agree with me here. I'm simply saying that if we take Hebrews 13:4 seriously, which teaches, "Marriage should be honored by all, and the marriage bed kept pure, for God will judge the adulterer and all the sexually immoral," then we should be consistent in our application. To me, I don't see how we can "honor marriage" while turning a blind eye to all the ways that professing Christians have devalued marriage. Heterosexuals do not get a pass when it comes to honoring marriage.

THE COST OF FOLLOWING CHRIST

Some may think that I am being unloving. I have no desire to be harsh, hurtful, or unloving to anyone. Yet, if God is love (1 John 4:8), has demonstrated His love in Christ to all of us (Rom. 5:8), and calls us to honor marriage (Heb. 13:4), then it must be that this command proceeds from the loving will of God for us. His commands are not heavy or burdensome (1 John 5:3). Furthermore, when Jesus defines what love to Him looks like, He tells us that it is embodied in keeping His commandments (John 14:21). If we are going to love others well, then our frame of reference must be following the God who defines Himself as love.

At this point, some may object and say that "such an action will irreparably harm my relationships and keep me from being able to share Christ with people in the future." I take this objection seriously. Furthermore, I appreciate the motive from which it proceeds. As I understand it, the person is trying to preserve the relationship so that future evangelistic attempts will not be harmed. My heart hurts for those in such situations, especially parents who face this kind of decision with their children. Let me share a few thoughts on this matter.

First, I believe it is important for all of us to remember that we are Christians first. Before I am a husband, a father, a pastor, or a professor, I am a Christian. My identity as a follower of Christ must shape every aspect of my life. Furthermore, we must realize that we will be the most pleasing husbands and wives, fathers and mothers, when we seek the kingdom of God first, before all other things. The best way for me to love my wife and children is to love God supremely. If I love them more than I love God, then I have turned them into idols. Only God is worthy of my supreme love. And in loving God foremost, I am called to submit myself to His righteousness. I cannot love God above all if I am also attempting to love the sins which Christ died to redeem me and others from. So, before we ever tackle the question of how best to relate to others, we must remember that our first priority is how we relate to God.

Once we have settled the matter of prioritizing our love for God above all, then, and only then, can we begin to work through what it would mean to love others well. In this case, loving others well would mean loving them in at least five different ways.[1] First, we are called to love boldly. Second Timothy 1:7 tells us that "the Spirit God gave us does not make us timid, but gives us power, love and self-discipline."

Much of what is directed on social media toward LGBTQ persons from self-identified evangelicals falls terribly short of the heartfelt compassion that Christians are called to be clothed in.

Some translations of this verse tell us that "God has not given us a spirit of fear," which the NIV translates as "does not make us timid." To love boldly or without fear is to love others with moral courage. If we love others, then we ought to love them enough to be truthful about what is pleasing and displeasing to God.

The second way that we are to love is to love compassionately. We see this in Colossians 3:12–13, which says, "Therefore, as God's chosen people, holy and dearly loved, clothe yourselves with compassion, kindness, humility, gentleness, and patience." Obviously, we are called to love with kindness, humility, gentleness, and patience as well from this verse, but I love the fact that compassion is one aspect of our Christian clothing. This is a "heartfelt compassion," which points to the genuineness of our affection for others. It is a love that is moved with mercy and tenderness. Much of what I see on social media directed toward LGBTQ persons from self-identified evangelicals falls terribly short of the heartfelt compassion that Christians are called to be clothed in.

The third way that we love is by loving truthfully. We have already seen this to a degree under the idea of loving boldly, but I think we need to repeat the insistence of Scripture on loving truthfully. One of the best examples of this sort of love is mentioned in Ephesians 4:15–16, where we read, "Instead, speaking the truth in love, we will grow to become in every respect the mature body of him who is the head, that is, Christ. From him the whole body, joined and held together by every supporting ligament, grows and builds itself up in love, as each part does its work." To be sure, the context for Ephesians 4:15–16 is love and truthful speech being spoken in the church of Jesus Christ. However, an implication of this passage would be that what motivates Christians to speak the truth is love for others. We must be mindful of the fact that there is a way to speak the truth that is not loving. Love must be what motivates us in our truth-speaking.

A fourth way to love is to love redemptively. We see this in the example of Christ in Titus 3:4–7, which tells us, "But when the kindness and love of God our Savior appeared, he saved us, not because of righteous things we had done, but because of his mercy. He saved us through the washing of rebirth and renewal by the Holy Spirit, whom he poured out on us generously through Jesus Christ our Savior, so that, having been justified by his grace, we might become heirs having the hope of eternal life." The coming of Christ was an expression of love and kindness with the aim to save sinners from their sin. If we do not tie our understanding of Christ's love to His redemptive purpose, then we will doubtlessly misunderstand it. Christ did not come to leave us the same, but to redeem us from our bondage to sin. In a similar way, our love toward others ought to be aimed at their redemption in the sense of them coming to Christ.

Finally, we ought to love patiently. Ephesians 4:2 tells us that we ought to strive to "be completely humble and gentle; be patient, bearing with one another in love." Again, the context here is in the church, but I believe it should also extend to our relationships outside of the church. Just as God was and is incredibly patient with us, we too ought to be patient with others, praying for them and working in the strength that God supplies to care for them and point them to God's grace in Jesus Christ. In all of this, we must see that loving others does not mean allowing the world to define what it means to "love," but rather, looking to God for our understanding of love as He has revealed it in His Word.

In the case of refusing to attend or support any wedding that undermines God's ideal of marriage, we are demonstrating that we will trust God with the impact that our decision makes to those who might not accept it. We can and must communicate that our decision is not rooted in hatred but rather love—love for God and love for them, which ultimately desires their good and God's glory. Yet, we recognize that it is impossible as a Christian to endorse a lifestyle or a decision that clearly contradicts God's desire for marriage. It would be unloving to do so.

CHAPTER EIGHT

What's in a Meal?— Welcoming My Gay Child and Their Partner at Thanksgiving

My child is gay and wants to bring their partner to Thanksgiving dinner. My child professes to be a Christian, but it is clear from their lifestyle that they are not following Christ. I love my child and do not want to estrange them from our family. At the same time, I do not approve of their lifestyle and am worried about how their presence at Thanksgiving could confuse my younger children. What should I do?"

Perhaps your family has already wrestled with a question like this. Perhaps you're a pastor and have already been asked for counsel. We live and minister in a world full of brokenness, which has resulted in moral confusion. Those asking such questions are grieving. They love their children dearly. They want to be good parents. But most of all, they want to honor God. They know that when they chose to follow Jesus, it might lead to conflict with some of their loved ones (Matt. 10:34–39).

Such moral dilemmas will not go away anytime soon. In fact, things will likely get more complex. But while things will not get easier to navigate, it is not as if moral dilemmas are particularly new. From Christianity's inception, starting with Jesus' own example, disciples of Jesus have had to wrestle with these types of questions. But God, in His grace, has not left us to wonder what His will is for us, even in complex situations in families like the one mentioned above.

IS EXCLUSION A CHRISTIAN CONCEPT?

Initially, some may read this scenario and wonder, "How is this even a question? Why wouldn't a Christian family welcome their child to a Thanksgiving dinner?" Others would take it a step further and question whether it is even right to ask the question of excluding someone. Didn't Jesus eat with sinners (Matt. 9:10–13; Luke 19:1–9)? More than likely, the proposed scenario and those like it come from certain interpretations and applications of passages like these:

> I wrote to you in my letter not to associate with sexually immoral people—not at all meaning the people of this world who are immoral, or the greedy and swindlers, or idolaters. In that case you would have to leave this world. But now I am writing to you that you must not associate with anyone who claims to be a brother or sister but is sexually immoral or greedy, an idolater or slanderer, a drunkard or swindler. Do not even eat with such people. (1 Cor. 5:9–11)

Second Thessalonians 3:6 and 14–15 reflect a similar message:

> In the name of the Lord Jesus Christ, we command you, brothers
> and sisters, to keep away from every believer who is idle and dis-
> ruptive and does not live according to the teaching you received
> from us. . . . Take special note of anyone who does not obey our
> instruction in this letter. Do not associate with them, in order
> that they may feel ashamed. Yet do not regard them as an enemy,
> but warn them as you would a fellow believer.

The similarity between these passages is not to suggest that the scenarios in these different churches are the same. But it shows that
the apostle Paul maintained a principle
of exclusion among the churches of Jesus
Christ. Paul did not invent this principle
out of thin air. As we will see, Jesus Himself commanded the practice of exclusion
as well.

If my child is constantly playing in the road, it would be unloving for me not to correct them. The same goes for our brothers and sisters in Christ's church who are playing with sin.

In Matthew 18:15–20, Jesus instructed
His disciples about handling unrepentant sinners in the context of the church.
Jesus begins with the aim of reconciling
a wayward brother or sister, saying, "If
your brother or sister sins, go and point
out their fault, just between the two of you. If they listen to you, you
have won them over." Instead of gossiping about someone, Jesus
commands His followers to take their concerns directly to the person
who has wandered away. This is an expression of love, not judgment.
The aim is restoration, not condemnation. If we suspend, for the moment, that "correction" is a "bad thing" or "judgmental thing," then it

is easy to see how such a practice is an act of love. As a parent, if my child is constantly playing in the road, it would be unloving for me not to correct them. The same goes for our brothers and sisters in Christ's church who are playing with sin.

Sadly, not every person responds the way that we hope they will respond to our attempts to restore them. So, Jesus continues, stating, "But if they will not listen, take one or two others along, so that 'every matter may be established by the testimony of two or three witnesses.'" Those who go with us in our effort to restore our wayward brother or sister ought to be actual witnesses to the waywardness, not people whom we have simply rallied to our restorative cause. We need to ensure that our restoration attempts are not tainted with gossip and slander.

If such restorative efforts are rebuffed a second time, Jesus says, "If they still refuse to listen, tell it to the church; and if they refuse to listen even to the church, treat them as you would a pagan or a tax collector." Notice that it is only as a final step that Jesus' followers move forward with bringing the offense to the church. Patience and wisdom should mark all such dealing. And the authority, which Jesus has delegated, belongs to the church as a gathered whole, not simply a few leaders within the church. Jesus speaks of this authority in the remaining verses, stating, "Truly I tell you, whatever you bind on earth will be bound in heaven, and whatever you loose on earth will be loosed in heaven. Again, truly I tell you that if two of you on earth agree about anything they ask for, it will be done for them by my Father in heaven. For where two or three gather in my name, there am I with them."

Though these last few verses in our passage are commonly used to support the idea of Christ's presence among a few gathered members (and it certainly does not exclude this reality), the passage is actually about the decision of the church to exclude a professing yet wayward believer from the fellowship of the church until they repent of their sin. The reason for this exclusion by the church is that the church plays a vital role in recognizing and affirming those who are part of the body of Christ. Through exclusion, the church says that this wayward believer has not repented of their sin, they have refused the accountability of Christ's body, and they have chosen to live in a manner contrary to Christ's teaching. And Jesus commands His church to exclude such professing "brothers and sisters" in the hope that they will repent, be restored, and ultimately be delivered from their hypocrisy. The aim is love.

As Jesus taught in Matthew 15:8, while people may make one confession with their lips, they are, nonetheless, presently denying that confession with their life. They are guilty of "honoring" Jesus with their lips while maintaining "hearts" that are far from him. Such *unrepentant* hypocrisy is not to be tolerated within the church of Jesus Christ. Please note the emphasis on *unrepentant*. Christians understand that we are saved and sustained by God's grace in Jesus Christ. Who among us is without sin? Who among us can claim on any given day to have perfectly reflected and conformed to God's perfect will? The only person present in our churches that can make such a claim is Christ Himself. According to Jesus, we need forgiveness like we need our daily bread (Matt. 6:9–13). Yet, this call to restore our wayward brothers and sisters in the church is aimed at restoring those who are falling away in sin and refusing to repent. Thus, as I hope it is clear by now, Paul's instruction in 1 Corinthians 5 and 2 Thessalonians 3, which we considered above, is firmly grounded in the teachings of Jesus, who, while welcoming all sinners without exception to come to Him (Matt. 11:28–30), also taught that those who come to Him must repent of their former sinful ways (Matt. 4:12–22).

We must maintain two truths about Jesus: Jesus was an inclusive Savior who welcomed everyone to come to Him, and yet, He was also an exclusive Savior who maintained certain expectations for those who decided to come to Him. He made a free offer to all (any could come), but the free offer was not cheap. The call to follow Jesus was open to anyone who would receive it, but it came with expectations. All are free to enter through the gate, but the gate is still narrow (Matt. 7:13–14).

What does this mean for us? We should not immediately rule out the possibility of exclusion because we have deemed it to be "unchristian." While exclusion is not a concept that our present society accepts (though a non-redemptive form of it can be observed in "cancel culture"), that does not mean that it is inherently an evil concept. Such exclusion is a form of discipline that aims to form the life of the unrepentant professing believer. And while discipline is not enjoyable, that does not mean it is not good or loving (Heb. 12:4–13). The aim of Christian exclusion was repentance and restoration. Exclusion from the people of God was a possibility that Jesus both affirmed and taught His disciples. We should not be surprised to see it in Paul's teachings.

But what bearing does such teaching have on our proposed scenario? How, if at all, does Jesus' teaching for the church inform Paul's instruction to the churches in Corinth and Thessalonica? Does it apply to our family gatherings over a meal? How can we reconcile Jesus' willingness to associate with sinners with the teaching that we find in Matthew 18, 1 Corinthians 5, and 2 Thessalonians 3? Should it be practiced in the case of our scenario?

THE DIFFERENCE BETWEEN THE CHURCH AND THE WORLD

One of the first things we need to see is that Jesus' instruction in Matthew 18 and Paul's instruction in 1 Corinthians 5 and 2 Thessalonians 3 regarding exclusion is that it appears in the context of the church of Jesus Christ. The church is the new covenant people of God, a community of professing believers in Jesus Christ. If you are a Christian, you have been baptized into the body of Christ, which symbolizes your trust in the life, death, burial, resurrection, and ascension of Jesus. It is through baptism that we, as believers, have publicly confessed our faith in Jesus Christ as our Lord and Savior. We have submitted to the lordship of Jesus over our entire life.

Because of our faith in Jesus, we, as believers, have been united to Him by the work of the Holy Spirit. We bear a new identity in Christ. The old has passed away, and the new creation has come (2 Cor. 5:17). And this is true of all members of the church, the body of Christ. If we are in Christ, we bear this new identity. For all the other identities that I'm sure you have, be that of a wife, husband, mother, father, an American, or an LSU football fan (Geaux Tigers!), when you became a Christian, all such identities were brought under the control of a new identity: the identity of being in Christ. And with this new identity in Christ comes new moral expectations. We are to live as those inhabited by Christ through the Holy Spirit as we are progressively being conformed to the image of Christ (Rom. 8:29). Much of the content found in the letters written to the New Testament churches focuses on forming this new identity in Christ. Believers are now part of a new community, the church, and thus, there was to be an observable break with the ways of the world. Being a part of God's family comes with certain familial obligations and expectations.

It is here that we start to get some clarity regarding how to reconcile Jesus and His free offer of the gospel, which welcomes all sinners to be forgiven and made new, with Jesus' instruction to the church to exclude unrepentant sinners from its fellowship. When relating to those who were *outside* of the church, those who had not professed faith in Him, Jesus did not shrink back. Jesus did not separate Himself from sinners. The apostle Paul maintained the same belief and practice, even telling the Corinthian believers that living a life of separation from sinners in the world would be impossible.

> *People in the world needed to hear the good news of God's grace in Christ. How would they ever hear if Christians withdrew from the world into some sort of holy huddle?*

Apparently, some people in Corinth had misunderstood Paul's instruction from a previous letter, but he sets the record straight in 1 Corinthians 5:9–10, "I wrote to you in my letter not to associate with sexually immoral people—not at all meaning the people of this world who are immoral, or the greedy and swindlers, or idolaters. In that case you would have to leave this world." Paul does not call believers to abandon the world to avoid sinners. In fact, his concern is not really with how people in the world are living, but rather how people within the church are living. People in the world needed to hear the good news of God's grace in Christ. How would they ever hear if Christians withdrew from the world into some sort of holy huddle? Such behavior contradicts Jesus' Great Commission, which tells us to "go into all the world"!

So, when reconciling Jesus' love for all sinners with His call to exclude sinners from the fellowship of the church, we must see that He is dealing with a particular group of sinners. Jesus is concerned, like Paul, with sinners who claim to be following Him but who refuse to repent of their sins and live in obedience to God's will for disciples. By definition, these are unrepentant sinners in the church of Jesus Christ. Such sinners needed to be warned, not welcomed. Welcoming such unrepentant sinners would have communicated a false message to them; namely, that it was okay for them to continue to live in rebellion against Christ while claiming to follow Him. But for sinners in the world who do not embrace Christ, they should be welcomed, not into the church as members per se, but to repent and believe in the good news of God's grace in Christ. All who were thirsty were welcomed to come and drink of the living water of Christ. All who were hungry were invited to feast on the bread of life in Christ.

When we interpret and apply the messages about exclusion in Matthew 18, 1 Corinthians 5, and 2 Thessalonians 3, we must remember that these are messages primarily given in the context of the church, and not a general principle about life in the world. The world needs the hope of the gospel. And as those who have experienced the power of the gospel, Christians ought to be faithfully and boldly living as salt and light, giving hope to a hopeless world.

HOW DO WE RELATE TO UNREPENTANT "CHRISTIANS" OUTSIDE OF THE CHURCH?

In many ways, keeping the context of the church and the world in mind will help us avoid misapplications of these texts about exclusion. However, in 1 Corinthians 5:11, Paul makes a statement that we need to clarify a little more. He writes, "But now I am writing to you that you must not associate with anyone who claims to be a brother or sister but is sexually immoral or greedy, an idolater or slanderer, a drunkard or swindler. Do not even eat with such people." It is this final sentence that has led to some debate among Christians about whether or not they are still allowed to have some sort of relationship with unrepentant Christians, which gets us back to a part of the dilemma we face in our proposed scenario about welcoming a child who is a professing believer yet living a lifestyle that is not in conformity with Christ.

On the surface, it appears that 1 Corinthians 5:11 rules out the possibility of having any relationship with unrepentant professing believers. For, as Paul says, "Do not even eat with such people." To sort through this situation, we must ask, "What did it mean to 'eat' or 'associate' with people in the first century? What did such an association communicate to the rest of the onlooking world?"

EATING AND DRINKING TOGETHER

In the first century, "eating and drinking together" was related to social bonding. Over a meal, friendships were formed and community identities were reinforced. We can see this in how the apostle Peter withdrew from eating with Gentile believers in Galatians 2. Out of fear of what other Jews would think about him, Peter stopped eating with Gentiles. The apostle Paul rebuked Peter for "not acting in line with the truth of the gospel" (Gal. 2:14). For Peter was more concerned with maintaining certain traditions related to table fellowship than living according to the standard of the gospel. Paul would not tolerate such disregard for the community-transforming power of the gospel. Why was eating with Gentiles such a big deal? Because it represented an erasure of certain boundary lines that threatened the identity of the Jewish community. In other words, it wasn't so much about Peter's personal preference but about maintaining an identity as a member of the Jewish community. But, according to Paul, the gospel of Jesus Christ had erased such boundaries by forming a new community of faith that included both Jews and Gentiles. And this community was the church of Jesus Christ.

In the first century, eating and drinking together was about more than hospitality. It sent a message to the world about who belonged to the community. If the Corinthian Christians continued to "eat with such people," it would have sent a message to the world that though these sinners are living contrary to the call of Christ, they still belong to the people of God. Jesus, as we saw in Matthew 18, and Paul, in 1 Corinthians 5, could not allow for such confusion to be promoted by the people of God. Continuing to associate with and affirm those who were blatantly living a lifestyle contrary to God's ways while still claiming to be a Christian would undermine one of the key roles that God had ordained the church to play in the world. How could the church be salt and light in the world if the church tolerated darkness? The church could not promote such confusion about who the people of God are and how they were to live in the world. This is what their meals, likely even in their private homes, would have communicated to the watching world in the first century. That's why Paul tells the Corinthian believers to avoid any scenario where their behavior, even meals, would communicate a message that was contrary to the gospel of Christ.

WHAT'S IN A MEAL?

So, what does this mean for our scenario from the beginning of the chapter? Do our meals together communicate an endorsement of the thoughts and behaviors of those who join us in our homes? Here is where I believe we encounter a significant point of difference between first-century Christians and present-day Christians in terms of the use of our houses and our meals, especially if we live in the West.

In the first century, houses were not only "the main place of living," but also the "place of worship" among Christians. Acceptance into one's home could have been regarded as acceptance into the Christian community. In our present day, however, our houses are rarely associated with our "place of worship." Furthermore, most of the meals in our homes do not connote acceptance into the religious community of the host. This means that while the exclusion of unrepentant professing believers in the context of the church should be practiced by all Christians concerned with following Jesus and Paul's instruction, it is unlikely that these passages would require us to stop relating to such people *outside of the church,* which would include meals in our homes.

However, it might be possible that there is a scenario where exclusion from eating or associating with unrepentant sinners would apply even in our homes. That scenario would be one in which such eating or association communicates to the person or the world that their presence in our homes or association with us means that they are "genuine Christians." If, however, we do not live in a culture where such eating and association connotes that such people are genuine Christians, but instead, is a form of hospitality or general kindness or an expression of familial relationship or common humanity, then I do not believe we are obligated to exclude people, even the unrepentant sinner. For conscience reasons, one might choose to do so, but I am not convinced that such an action is required by Paul's instruction in 1 Corinthians 5:11.

There are times we need to maintain and nurture relationships to love people and exhort them to turn back to Christ, especially our children. In fact, I would say that we ought to make a special effort to invite them into our lives so that the light of the gospel might pierce the darkness and lead them to repentance and faith in Christ.

BUT WHAT ABOUT MY OTHER CHILDREN?

While we have established that meals and homes among first-century Christians functioned differently than our own, we haven't dealt with the question of how welcoming unrepentant professing believers might impact our other children. Some will doubtless think that such a concern represents "protectionism" or "isolationism." As you have likely heard people say, "You cannot protect your kids from everything," or "I don't want to shelter my children from the world." Before we address the specific question in view, I want to address these common objections.

The idea that parents cannot or should not "protect" or "shelter" their children from certain sins in the world is not only a poor parenting philosophy, it also requires a poor reading of Scripture. Take, for instance, the book of Proverbs. Much of the book, though not all, is written from the perspective of a father to a son. Any fair reading of the book of Proverbs cannot help but conclude that part of a parent's role is to warn their children to avoid certain sins and situations. Parents do not have to allow their children to get burned by a campfire to warn them that the fire is hot. Any parent allowing their child to get burned to "teach them a valuable lesson" is being abusive and not loving. From my experience, these objections related to "protecting" or "sheltering" a child come from a parental philosophy that is more informed by the world than the wisdom of God. Honestly, if parents do not have some sort of responsibility to "protect" or "shelter" their children, then what are they even doing? So, parents, it is not only okay but natural and good to desire to protect your children from the destructiveness and deceitfulness of sin in the world.

But protecting and sheltering are not enough. When "protecting" and "sheltering" are not coupled with the gospel and intentional discipleship, all we end up with are children who know the world is dangerous but do not know how to live in it. Furthermore, we end up with children who think that they are "okay with God" because they are "not like those other kids." If we are not careful, we can unwittingly teach our children that the "kingdom of God" belongs to the "good people," but such a message contradicts the gospel of God's grace. I saw and experienced this firsthand while growing up in a Christian school. I'm not saying there is something wrong with Christian schools. In fact, I'm grateful for so much of my time in this particular school, but I want to share an example of how we must be careful in what we communicate to our children.

While attending a Christian elementary school, I won the "Best Christian Example" award. If memory serves correctly, I won the award twice (my mom probably still has the certificate). The award was given to a few children who demonstrated exemplary conduct in the classroom. The main problem, I wasn't even a Christian! God did not save me until I was seventeen years old. Was I well-behaved? Compared to others, probably, but I was also deceitful. I figured out a way to take the Keith Green and 4Him cassette tapes (google it) that my mom bought me at the religious bookstore and record over them with songs off the radio. While my boombox looked like I was jamming to Keith Green's "Grace By Which I Stand," I was really listening to Snoop Dogg's "Gin and Juice." I would even call the request line (again, google it) at KMJJ and request these songs to be ready to record them off the radio.

But you know what? I still had that "Best Christian Example" award, which assured me that I must be a Christian because it seemed like I behaved well. I was as lost as the next person, yet when the essence of what it means to be a "Christian" is measured solely by outward behavior instead of inward affections that depend on the supernatural work of the Holy Spirit, we can, even unknowingly, end up manipulating our children into acting right while their hearts are still far from God.

While kids raised in Christian homes might think and act differently than other kids, they are still sinners in need of God's mercy. It's fine to teach your children how to sit quietly in a worship service, how to have good manners, how to find Bible verses quickly, and how to answer the catechism, but these things in and of themselves do not change their hearts. Only the Holy Spirit can do that as He accompanies the gospel of God's grace in Christ that we teach them regularly through our own words and actions. This means that while our parenting should certainly include moral in-struction and formative discipline, it must also be marked by a per-sistent prayer to God to do what only He can do in the hearts of our children. At the end of the day, we must realize that while we can try to "shelter" and "protect" them from the world, we cannot shelter or protect them from their own hearts, which God's Word teaches us are "deceitful above all things" (Jer. 17:9). Our children need a supernatural work of God's grace!

What does this mean for our situation where we have younger, impressionable children?

When we realize that our children need the gospel just like every-one else, I believe we are freed from fear to love others and live faith-fully in this world as those who know that our only hope is in Christ.

Our children are not saved by avoiding sinful people, because they are sinful people too. And the hope for your children is the same hope for the rest of the world. The sooner we understand this, the sooner we will be able to love others boldly in Christ!

So, what does this mean for our situation where we have younger, impressionable children and an older sibling who is a professing believer yet is living in open rebellion against Christ? Given what we understand about everyone's need for the gospel of Christ, I believe the opportunity to host that older sibling in the presence of the younger children is a chance to show our children how to love others with the redemptive compassion that we see exemplified in Jesus.

The reality is that in our proposed scenario, the older sibling needs to be reminded of the grace, mercy, kindness, and holiness of Christ. For, as Paul wrote in Romans 2:4, "God's kindness is intended to lead [us] to repentance." When we meet with those who need to repent, we, as followers of Christ, are to be conduits of God's kindness, praying that God would use our presence and persistence in the lives of those who have strayed to turn them back to God. The wayward older child needs to repent just as the younger child needs to repent. And how can we expect such repentance to take place in their lives if we remove our gospel witness from them?

If we carry this mentality into our relationships, especially with our children who have strayed, and we explicitly teach our other children why we are engaged in this behavior and why they need the gospel too, I believe we have not only modeled a life that reflects Christ's concern, but we have shown them what it means to live as disciples in the world (John 17:14–19). As a Christian parent, I cannot imagine a better lesson to teach our children.

When faced with the moral dilemma of how to love our wayward children well without confusing other children or compromising our faithfulness to Christ, as long as we are not affirming people in their rebellion against Christ or deceiving them into believing that they are living as genuine believers, I believe we are free and should maintain our relationships with them. This includes but is not limited to welcoming them to our table, having them in our homes, and generally showing kindness and love. I believe this is the way of Jesus that we are called to follow as salt and light in the world.

To be sure, this does not mean those unrepentant professing believers will always agree with our approach to these relationships. Many times, such people will not accept anything except a full-throated affirmation, acceptance, and celebration of their lifestyles. As followers of Christ, we cannot affirm the rebellion that He died to deliver us from in this world. We must be faithful to obey Christ above all, who commands us to love God above everything and everyone while loving others as ourselves.

We have been dealing with some heavy issues, as we must be prepared to respond to the real-life situations we are being confronted with. The world may seem dark—and it is—and yet our Lord is the Light of the World. At this point, we'll return to our biblical and theological framework that undergirds everything we've been discussing and be refreshed by the promise of what's ahead.

CHAPTER NINE

Exploring the Biblical-Theological Framework Four

CREATION REGAINED: "Behold, I Saw a New Heaven and New Earth"

At this point in my pastoral ministry, I have officiated far more funerals than weddings. Maybe this is because the first two churches that I served as lead pastor were what some people would call "revitalization works." Such churches typically have a relatively long history and a stable core membership of committed but older church members. As the communities around these churches change, the churches often begin to decline for various reasons. But there is still great gospel work to be done in these churches and in such communities.

I cherish many of the memories of those days. They taught me something about pastoral ministry. They taught me how to preach funerals for believers, for unbelievers, for friends, and for family members. I was often asked to lead a graveside service for most of those funerals.

One of my favorite truths to remind people of was the coming resurrection of the dead in Christ upon His return. When possible, I would usually point to all the gravesites around us. Many of the markers around us had Bible verses on them, like "to live is Christ, to die is gain," or "gone to be with Jesus." Even while standing in the middle of a field of death and loss, hope remained. So, as I pointed to the graves around us, I would tell the family and friends who gathered with us that one day, this field of death and loss would burst forth with resurrection life when Christ returned. One day, graveyards would look more like family reunions. I believe this is one of the reasons why so many churches used to maintain their own graveyards on their grounds. It wasn't just because it provided a service to their congregation; it was also an image of hope that we would all be gathered to Him together at the same time.

Over the last decade of serving as a lead pastor, the sermons that I have received the most (by far) positive responses to are sermons about God's new creation. Sometimes these sermons deal with the topic of heaven, or the intermediate state between death and the resurrection, or the hope of the resurrection at Jesus' return. People are hungry for hope on the other side of this life, and Christians have every reason to be filled with such hope when we consider what Christ has done for us.

There is coming a day when death itself will be fully and finally defeated for Christ's people.

As we know, while our present experience of salvation is amazing, we still face and feel the consequences of sin all around us. I don't make a single hospital visit without being struck by the brokenness in this world. This created world, as Paul put it in Romans 8:19–21, groans for redemption, a return to Eden—but actually for something better than Eden. This is what Christ has accomplished as the "firstfruits" of the resurrection (1 Cor. 15:20–28). What Adam lost for all humanity, Christ regains for His new humanity, those who have put their trust in Him.

There is coming a day when death itself will be fully and finally defeated for Christ's people (1 Cor. 15:26). You may ask, "Why do you say, 'for Christ's people'?" This is a good but probably uncomfortable question for some. I say "for Christ's people," because of how John speaks of the return of Christ in Revelation 20. According to Revelation 20–22, when Christ returns, those who had placed their trust in Him while living on this earth will be resurrected to meet Him in the air as He descends to rule over the earth. The apostle Paul speaks of this in 1 Thessalonians 4:13–18, saying,

> Brothers and sisters, we do not want you to be uninformed
> about those who sleep in death, so that you do not grieve like
> the rest of mankind, who have no hope. For we believe that
> Jesus died and rose again, and so we believe that God will bring
> with Jesus those who have fallen asleep in him. According to the
> Lord's word, we tell you that we who are still alive, who are left
> until the coming of the Lord, will certainly not precede those
> who have fallen asleep. For the Lord himself will come down
> from heaven, with a loud command, with the voice of the arch-
> angel and with the trumpet call of God, and the dead in Christ
> will rise first. After that, we who are still alive and are left will be

caught up together with them in the clouds to meet the Lord in the air. And so we will be with the Lord forever. Therefore encourage one another with these words.

Paul wrote these words to encourage the church in Thessalonica who had questions about their fellow Christians who died before Christ returned. They wanted to know what to do with this seeming dilemma. Some scholars suggest that the early church expected Jesus to return at any moment, and that they would be spared death. Yet, when believers started to die and Christ hadn't returned yet, they worried that something was wrong. Paul explains that these believers, though dead, will still conquer death. Death doesn't get the final word. For, just as Jesus was raised from the dead, so also everyone who has placed their trust in Him in this life will also be raised when He returns.

CREATION REGAINED

What will this new creation be like? Given that our experience of this new creation is a future event, we do not know all the specific details. But just because we do not have an exhaustive knowledge of the new creation doesn't mean that we cannot have some true knowledge of what it will be like.

For starters, we will be like Christ. We are told in 1 John 3:2–3, "Dear friends, now we are children of God, and what we will be has not yet been made known. But we know that when Christ appears, we shall be like him, for we shall see him as he is. All who have this hope in him purify themselves, just as he is pure." There is still a mystery here, but we at least know that we will be like Christ. Given what the rest of Scripture says about the believer's resurrection (1 Cor. 15), we know that this means we will receive a new, incorruptible, immortal body that will never be subject to sin or death again. But in order for this to be the case, God must deal with the brokenness of creation. Hence, a new—or as some describe it, a renewed—creation. John also makes this clear in the final chapters of the book of Revelation where we read that God "will wipe every tear from their eyes. There will be no more death or mourning or crying or pain, for the old order of things has passed away" (Rev. 21:4).

Imagine such a world! A world with no more death, no more tears, no more cancer diagnoses, no more abuse, no more pain, no more sin. It sounds a lot like what Eden was intended to be, and if you read Revelation 20–22 closely, you'll start to understand why. At the beginning of Revelation 22, we see a long-lost image from Genesis 1–3 reappear. It's the "Tree of Life," which Adam and Eve were banished from when they rebelled against God and were expelled from the garden of Eden. As John brings the greatest story ever told to a close (which is really a new beginning), he wants us to see how everything that we lost because of sin is regained in Christ, but in a much better way. Creation itself is regained as God deals with rebellion through judgment and welcomes His people into His presence forever. As John writes about the believer's inheritance, "They will see his face, and his name will be on their foreheads," which is a sign of Christ's commitment to us as those who belong to Him. John continues, "There will be no more night. They will not need the light of a lamp or the light of the sun, for the Lord God will give them light. And they will reign for ever and ever" (Rev. 22:4–5).

This is how God makes everything right. He decrees judgments for those who did not accept Christ's work on their behalf as the atoning sacrifice for sin, and He welcomes those who did accept Christ's work, having their sins atoned for by the blood of Jesus. This is what makes the good news not only for now but forever. Evil is dealt with finally and righteousness reigns forever. God is vindicated as the Judge of all the earth who always does what is right.

We've been carefully developing a biblical framework for practical responses to some of the most challenging questions of our times. In the next two chapters, we'll consider another: gender dysphoria.

But first, as we reflect on the consummation of the salvation that Christ has secured for His people as creation itself is regained and redeemed, here are a couple of questions to ponder:

1. How does the hope of the believer's full and final redemption in Christ inform our perspective about our present trials in this life?
2. How should our thoughts about the new creation impact the way we relate to our present use and enjoyment of creation?

CHAPTER TEN

"My Daughter Believes She's My Son"— Gender Dysphoria in the Home

Growing up, one of my brothers was torn about what he wanted to be when he grew up. Apparently, it was between being a hook truck driver or a German shepherd. To my parents' relief, the German shepherd part didn't work out, but neither did the hook truck driver. He ended up doing something different with his life, but the fact they knew he was just a kid with a vivid imagination to think he could be a dog didn't worry them too much. He would grow out of it. This is just what kids do, or at least this is what we once thought as a society.

Today, though, many parents are facing increasing pressure to embrace a view of the world that is contrary to God's design for humanity. In particular, many parents are facing the issue of gender dysphoria and gender identity issues with their children. And for parents that are not dealing with these issues in their own homes, they are certainly encountering them in broader society. It may be in their local sports league or maybe in their classroom at school or on social media, where so much of the sexual revolution has influenced the next generation. Gender dysphoria refers to a "deep sense of unease and distress that may occur when your biological sex does not match your gender identity."[1] If you are not familiar with what I'm referring to here, imagine a biological male experiencing a "deep sense of unease and distress" about being male and feeling as though he should be a female. Sometimes this unease and distress is captured in the phrase "born in the wrong body." For people who experience gender dysphoria, something feels out of sorts with who they believe they are (gender identity) and their physical embodiment (biological sex). How should parents respond when their child expresses such feelings to them?

LISTEN CLOSELY

First, parents should listen closely to their children. Do not be dismissive or angry at them for being willing to speak to you about their struggle. I believe that this principle is taught in passages like James 1:19, which tells us, "Everyone should be quick to listen, slow to speak and slow to become angry." I realize these conversations can be uncomfortable, but don't allow the discomfort to control your response. As parents, we want our children to know that they are speaking with someone who regards them and their struggles with seriousness and love.

Sometimes parents are tempted to start responding to their children before they are even finished speaking, which undermines the integrity of the relationship. I know that I have been guilty of this with my children. They will bring me a complaint or a concern about something at school or in the home, and instead of listening to them, I begin to speak over them. On a few occasions, my children have told me, "You're not even listening to me!" I wish I could say I have always responded well to their protests, but that is not true. If I'm being honest, sometimes I spoke over them because I was uncomfortable with what I was hearing from them. An unwillingness to listen to one's child often leads to provoking them to anger, which God's Word prohibits (Eph. 6:4 ESV). Instead of provoking them to anger with our response, our aim ought to be to listen well so that we might better understand their struggle, and then respond appropriately with "the training and instruction of the Lord."

Furthermore, for parents in this situation, do not listen to the voice of shame that you will likely wrestle with in these moments. As parents, you want to cultivate the type of relationship with your children where they will not be afraid to speak with you about the things that they are struggling with in life. Again, I have not always done this well, but it is something that I strive for with my own children. If my kids are struggling, I want them to know that I am a safe person to speak with. They don't have to fear my response. My wife and I are here to help them. I assure my kids that we will get through whatever it is that they are facing. We are for our kids, and I would encourage you to be as well.

Parents, you do not have to have all the answers to every question or struggle that your child faces. Often the best way is to sit down with a counselor who understands the dynamics of the struggles and who is also committed to God's Word.

A great illustration of this response can be found in the parable of the lost son in Luke 15:11–32. In that parable, a son demands his part of the inheritance from his (still living) father. The father grants the son's request, and the son runs headlong into the far country, squandering his inheritance. The son eventually comes to his senses and returns to his father, but not without being weighed down by shame. The father could have responded by saying, "You got what you asked for, but you no longer have a place here."

This, however, is not how the father responded. Instead of feeling shame at the son's return, the father took off running toward the son as he saw him approaching home. He embraced him in love and for-giveness, celebrating his return. Now, I'm fully aware that this passage is teaching us about more than a father's embrace of a prodigal son. Yet, we should not miss the comfort and hope that this story provides to parents whose children have run from God. Jesus uses a story about a father's love and embrace of a repentant son to teach us something about God's love, which we would do well to remember when we are caring for our own children.

SHED STRICT STEREOTYPES

As we walk with our children through these struggles about gen-der and sexuality, we need to be sure that we listen well to what has prompted their crisis. In some cases, the best way to address these concerns will be to sit down with a counselor who understands the dynamics of the struggles and is also committed to the same vision of gender and sexuality that God's Word reveals. Parents, you do not have to have all the answers to every question or struggle that your child faces. Do not laden yourself with that kind of burden. Fur-thermore, I would hope that you are part of a church that can walk alongside you in prayer and support (Gal. 6:2). If you are not, find a church that will. Parenting is not a journey to undertake alone.

After listening to your child, you may find that their struggle with gender dysphoria is more related to confusion about what it means to be a boy or a girl in the world. There is a lot of unnecessary confusion in our world about what it means to bear God's image and reflect our uniqueness. For about four years, I lived and pastored in a rural part of south Arkansas. Hunting and fishing were just a part of our lives. If we follow the stereotypes of gender, then we wouldn't expect to find many young women being interested in hunting and fishing, but that could not have been further from the truth in Arkansas. In fact, many of the women in the community killed more trophy bucks than some of the men. Yet what was interesting was that those same women didn't regard themselves as men simply because they were interested in things that were stereotypically male activities. In other words, just because they didn't fit the stereotype of being a woman didn't mean that they were doubting whether they were truly women.

It just shows that we need to be careful to not allow narrow or strict stereotypes of what it means to be a male or female to sway our children from embracing who God has made them to be in the world. It is very likely that a young boy who prefers singing over sports might feel that something is wrong with him because his peers do not have the same interest, but we need to fight against such a vision. The same goes with our daughters. If our girls prefer sports to Barbies, that is okay. Don't fret about it! Their interest in the more rough and tumble aspects of life do not mean that they are less of a girl. And don't let others tell them that either! When we are committed to listening to our children, we may very well find that the problem they are struggling with is related to a misunderstanding that has been foisted upon them.

Now, this is not to suggest that there are no differences between boys and girls. Instead, it is to say that those differences are related more to their embodied existences than their fleeting preferences for athletics or the arts. Our boys are boys because they are biological males, which means that their bodies are ordered according to God's purpose for males in the world. And the same goes for our girls. In time, these differences become exceedingly apparent as their DNA and hormones progress according to God's plan for males and females.

THE TRANS QUESTION

I believe that under no circumstance should a parent allow their child to "transition" either socially, hormonally, or surgically. Any professional advocating such action to "treat" gender dysphoria should be rejected. Such "transitions" cause far more harm than allowing time and physical maturing to work itself out in their children. In fact, several studies have shown that many children who experience gender dysphoria see it resolve on its own without any treatment.

Consider this statement from Dr. Debra Soh, a neuroscientist who is internationally regarded as a sex researcher: "Across all eleven long-term studies ever done on gender dysphoric children, between 60 and 90 percent desist by puberty. Desistence refers to the phenomenon of gender dysphoria remitting."[2] This idea of "desistence" is not popular among gender activists, but you must be aware of these studies as a parent helping a child wrestle through their feelings of dysphoria. Making life-altering, irreversible decisions to a child struggling with gender dysphoria is not healthcare, nor is it consistent with a Christian view of humanity created in God's image. We must reject the warped counsel of those who would encourage us to maim our children to address a psychological condition. Furthermore, so-called gender affirmation treatments have been demonstrated to not result in better mental health or long-term happiness. In fact, the opposite is true. "Persons with transsexualism, after sex reassignment, have considerably higher risks for mortality, suicidal behaviour, and psychiatric morbidity than the general population."[3]

So, parents, be patient, listen well, pray for your children. Get them solid Christian, professional counseling, and instruct them in the truth without anger or frustration. Don't let the shifting sands and blowing winds of society influence how you train your child up in the fear and the admonition of the Lord. If, in listening to your children, you find that they are encountering influences among friends, schoolmates, teachers, counselors, administrators, social media personalities, or even family members, remove those influences as fast as possible. This might mean changing schools or even homeschooling for a season. It might mean showing up at a school board meeting to voice your concerns. It might mean taking away their smartphone or using an app that monitors their online activity. It might mean a whole host of things, but this is your child we are talking about. Don't worry about what other people think of you. Care for your children first. God gave them to you as a stewardship. Care for them well!

THE GOSPEL FOR PARENTS

If parenting has taught me anything, it's that it is easy to be consumed by guilt. I never really thought of myself as a selfish person until I got married. Then, after my wife and I had kids, I realized just how selfish I can be. Parenting regularly exposes my need for the grace of God, not only for my children but for me as well. When it comes to difficult scenarios like the one posed in this chapter, Christian parents desperately need to be reminded of the promises of the gospel of Jesus Christ.

For starters, parents, we need to realize that while we have a responsibility to sow the seed of the gospel in our children's hearts and even water that seed over time, ultimately God is the one who makes that seed grow. Paul spoke of this in 1 Corinthians 3:6, saying, "I planted the seed, Apollos watered it, but God has been making it grow." We need to be reminded of the "but Gods" of the Bible. We are called to do some things, but there are other things that only God can do. We can pray, teach, love, play, discipline, laugh, model, plead, and a host of other things, but we do not have the power to give our children spiritual life or rescue them from every struggle they have. But God can. God loves our children more than we do. He is more faithful than we are. And most importantly, He is more powerful as well.

These are the types of promises that we must cling to. In and of ourselves, we are not sufficient for the things that we have been called to. And while that may sound like "bad news," trust me, it's not. It is good to be reminded that we are not God. While we are not sufficient, He is. As Ephesians 3:20 tells us, He is "able to do immeasurably more than all we ask or imagine, according to his power that is at work within us." What a promise! God is able to do even more than we "ask or imagine." While activists will tell us that our children's struggles are their destinies, we must remember who our God is!

THE GOSPEL FOR CHILDREN

In remembering who our God is, we must not forget the power of the gospel to transform our children. The gospel is still the power of God unto salvation. Our God can change and deliver us and our children from every struggle we face. As such, gender dysphoria, while a result of sin in the world (like all mental illnesses), is not a child's greatest enemy. A child's greatest enemy is being outside of Christ. Thus, while a parent might be overwhelmed by the thought of their child being transgender or struggling with gender dysphoria, such a struggle is a manifestation of the root issues of sin, which infect all of us in this fallen world. I am not dismissing the struggle, nor suggesting that there are simple fixes.[4] But the gospel deals with our root issues, whatever they might be in our lives or our children's lives.

You might be tempted to lose hope, but look to Christ. Our hope is a living hope: Christ crucified, buried, and raised from the dead. He speaks life where there appears to be no hope for life. He works miracles where others have said "there is simply no way." Don't buy the lie that your children are beyond the saving hand of God through Christ (Isa. 59:1). Hope in the One who has conquered the grave itself! If God can conquer death, surely He is more than able to conquer the trials that we face in this life. God is for you, not against you.

Whatever situation you may be facing with loved ones, dwell on and find hope in this passage.

> What, then, shall we say in response to these things? If God is for us, who can be against us? He who did not spare his own Son, but gave him up for us all—how will he not also, along with him, graciously give us all things? Who will bring any charge against those whom God has chosen? It is God who justifies. Who then is the one who condemns? No one. Christ Jesus who died—more than that, who was raised to life—is at the right hand of God and is also interceding for us. Who shall separate us from the love of Christ? Shall trouble or hardship or persecution or famine or nakedness or danger or sword? As it is written:
>
> > "For your sake we face death all day long; we are considered as sheep to be slaughtered."

No, in all these things we are more than conquerors through him who loved us. For I am convinced that neither death nor life, neither angels nor demons, neither the present nor the future, nor any powers, neither height nor depth, nor anything else in all creation, will be able to separate us from the love of God that is in Christ Jesus our Lord. (Rom. 8:31–39)

CHAPTER ELEVEN

The Transgender Man Sitting in the Third Pew— Gender Dysphoria in the Church

Visiting a church for the first time can be uncomfortable. Years ago, while on vacation with my whole family, my brother and I slipped away on a Sunday morning to a church in the area for worship. We intentionally went to a church outside of our tradition to see what it was like. The church was warm and welcoming, but they approached corporate worship differently. They had a prophecy microphone and enthusiastically spoke in tongues without an interpreter. While these things were not new to me, they were definitely not part of my everyday experience in worship. But I was simply not ready for what happened next.

I was still a pretty immature teenager then, so when the flag-wavers and interpretive dancers made their way to the front of the auditorium, you can probably imagine how I responded. There are few things as hard as holding in a laugh when you are in church. I just hoped that no one would come to talk to me. I was really uncomfortable. Needless to say, we didn't make it back to that church the next time we were in that area, but I'll never forget how it made me feel. I felt out of place. There was no explanation regarding why things were being done, just my experience of those things happening.

IN THE GATHERING

I am older now and, I would hope, more mature. But that feeling of not belonging while visiting that church sticks with me. As I have aged and studied God's Word more closely, I've come to realize that "feeling comfortable" or "sensing that I belong" is not exactly why the church gathers week in and week out on Sunday mornings. While I still believe it is important for churches to practice hospitality, our goal is not for everyone who attends to immediately feel as though they are the reason why the church gathers. The church gathers to worship the living and reigning Christ. And in the process of worshiping Christ, not everyone may feel like they belong, at least not initially. But is this a biblical principle?

One of my favorite passages of Scripture is found in 1 Corinthians 14:24–25. It says, "But if an unbeliever or an inquirer comes in while everyone is prophesying, they are convicted of sin and are brought under judgment by all, as the secrets of their hearts are laid bare. So they will fall down and worship God, exclaiming, 'God is really among you!'" I doubt that many of you will use this passage of Scripture in your family Christmas cards, but the passage is an essential reminder to us about why we gather together and how God works through His church.

As the Spirit of God moves among the people of God, we worship the Lord in Spirit and in truth. This is our aim when we gather. We meet so that Christ might be magnified by His body as each member builds the other members up through the exercising of their spiritual gifts. Yet, this is not to the complete exclusion of those who have not yet trusted in Christ. As the passage notes, there may be times when "an unbeliever or an inquirer" gathers alongside the members of Christ's body. Obviously, then, we ought not be closed to the idea of such people being in our worship gatherings. Paul, inspired by the Holy Spirit, expects that there might be a time when this happens. Thus, we ought to anticipate it. We ought to even encourage it. But that should not change what we do as God's people. For, as God's people do what He has called them to do, God moves in our midst.

In the case of the Corinthian church, this is what Paul expected to happen. God's people would obey Him, and He would move among them. And in the cases where unbelievers or inquirers were present, God would work through His people to bring them under conviction of sin and declare that God was truly among them.

Recently, I have watched some professing Christians on social media claim that we could (or should) prohibit certain people from attending church. Most of them talked about people who were transgender. And to be fair, some also mentioned people who dressed in drag, which some would classify as different than transgender. These people asserted that churches should prohibit the attendance of transgender people or people dressed in drag. If I were to give such claims the benefit of the doubt, then I would assume that they are trying to apply the passages of Scripture that deal with adorning ourselves in modest apparel. I appreciate the attempt to take the Bible seriously and apply it consistently, but I find such appeals to such passages lacking.

It's good for churches to have certain expectations of what's appropriate attire for corporate worship. This is certainly true in the case of someone arriving dressed in drag, which is performative and inappropriate for church. However, a different situation would be an unsuspecting transgender person who arrives at your church. Maybe they thought that your church would affirm their lifestyle. Maybe they thought it wouldn't be an issue. Or maybe they thought that this church in their community could help them with a situation they were facing in their life. But for whatever reason, assuming that their presence is not to incite some sort of protest or disrupt the service, I believe churches should be open to receiving all who are sincerely interested in attending.

Churches are under no obligation to entertain foolishness or blasphemy in the name of hospitality. I remember a few instances in which I either had a role in escorting individuals out of a church building or having a very uncomfortable conversation that led to people leaving of their own accord. One was a man who stood up during our service and screamed "God is dead," another was a woman who was panhandling during the service, and another was denying someone's request to serve as a volunteer in our children's ministry after learning that the person recently had been released from prison after serving time for child abuse.

Why should the church receive those sincerely searching? Let's start by considering why the church exists at all.

These, though, were exceptional situations, and I should interject here that we followed up as best we could, with mixed results. Most people in these communities who needed help received it without any issues. We welcomed them into the church and did everything within our ability to make sure they knew that we wanted them with us. Those who wanted real help received it. Their need was sincere, and we did what we could to help. When people are sincerely searching, the church needs to be willing to receive them. Furthermore, I do not mention these examples to suggest that a transgender guest poses some threat to the church but rather to demonstrate that the idea that "everyone is welcome" is always a qualified invitation.

Why should the church receive those sincerely searching? Let's start by considering why the church exists at all. In Ephesians 3:20–21, Paul tells us that the church exists to glorify God, which means magnifying God by showing others what He is really like through our words and deeds. And, as we have already considered in previous chapters, our God is a seeking God. He comes to seek and save that which was lost (Luke 19:10)! He comes for those who are sick and needy (Luke 5:31–32). Thus, if the church is going to glorify God, then it must welcome those who are sincerely searching, even if their life is a complete mess when we meet them. And, if we are being honest with ourselves, this is how we all were before God changed our lives by the power of His gospel!

PRACTICAL MATTERS

But what would welcoming a transgender guest look like practically in a local church? What about things like bathrooms or gender-organized ministries (men's ministry, women's ministry)? How can a church do this well in love without compromising truth? I believe our answers to these types of questions must keep in mind the church's purpose.

Namely, the church exists to glorify God, which would entail not only equipping church members with a biblical view of sexuality and gender but also forming and enforcing policies and procedures in the church that reflect biblical truth. Churches are forming the spirituality of their members not only through what they say but also through what they do.

Take, for instance, the question of bathroom usage in the local church. What should a church do if someone who identifies as transgender visits the church and wants to use the bathroom of their preferred gender? Here's how I would counsel a church in this situation. First, churches should be proactive in creating restroom usage policies that affirm biblical truth regarding biological sex and gender. Second, they should formulate such policies in a manner that compassionately communicates the dignity of all attendees. In other words, these policies are for everyone. Churches have expectations for everyone, not just their guests. I doubt that this point will be controversial, since most churches have certain expectations depending on the situation. At every church I have pastored, we had security protocols for our children's ministry. Volunteers had to be background-checked and trained. Certain areas of the building were off-limits to those who were not volunteering. We had volunteer-to-kid ratios to ensure accountability and safety. Such expectations should not surprise or anger anyone who actually cares about the safety and well-being of others.

But how can a church implement these types of training and poli-

One of the best ways churches can prepare is by organizing hospitality or security teams to help direct guests based on their needs. Ideally, such teams should consist of church members of both genders.

cies? One of the best ways churches can prepare for such situations is by organizing hospitality or security teams to help direct guests based on their needs. Ideally, such teams should consist of church members of both genders. The guests' needs could range from the location of the bathrooms to the date and time of certain Bible studies. Obviously, this will require that hospitality and security teams be trained to deal with different situations that might arise in the church. The training should be clear, compassionate, and convictional. Furthermore, the training should be aimed at helping guests while not minimizing the reality of threats that may present themselves.

I'm not suggesting that guests of any gender or sexual orientation or who struggle with gender identity present a specific kind of threat in every situation. That would be a foolish conclusion that breeds unwarranted suspicions about every person who walks into our churches. However, it would be equally foolish not to have a plan to address issues that might arise, even issues that have nothing to do with the current matters the church faces regarding gender and sexuality in society. Does this feel messy? Yes. But when sinners come together in the church, things often get messy. Churches must heed Jesus' instructions to be "wise as serpents and innocent as doves" (Matt. 10:16 ESV). We should have no desire to cause undue offense to anyone we encounter, but we also must recognize our obligation to care for those that God has entrusted to us.

Another practical way that a church can proactively address this scenario is by posting its stated policy on the bathroom doors and/ or creating unisex, single-occupancy restrooms that accommodate all attendees. Admittedly, the problem with simply posting a policy is that compliance with the policy depends on the willingness of attendees to adhere to the policies. This is why, if I had to pick a preference here, I would suggest having a unisex, single-occupancy restroom that is available to all guests.

How should church leadership respond and advise a transgender individual who is biologically male wishing to partake in a women's Bible study? This scenario should likely be handled case by case with significant input from the Bible study leaders and their current group members. If a group of women in a Bible study chose to include the transgender person in their study for the sake of sharing the gospel or helping the person work through what it looks like to repent and follow Jesus, it would seem like such scenarios would be biblically permissible but not biblically mandated.

If, however, the transgender individual is a professed believer with no interest in submitting to Christ's lordship over their gender and biological sex, such a scenario would undermine the clarity of gospel repentance and risk affirming them in a lifestyle that is contrary to God's will for disciples of Christ. Another option would be for women who are willing to meet with the transgender individual in a different setting to study the Bible, so long as there is clarity regarding gospel repentance and God's will for disciples of Christ in matters of gender and biological sex.

Churches will require wisdom to produce and teach through various kinds of policies and scenarios.

With that said, no women's Bible study group should be forced to include someone of the opposite sex in their meetings, nor should they be made to feel as though their exclusion of a transgender person from their group is in violation of the command to love one's neighbor. Love of one's neighbor does not include affirming another person's self-perception. If a women's Bible study group chose to allow the transgender individual to participate in the group, they should do so with wisdom and self-awareness of this situation with the intention of discipling the individual to faithfully follow Christ. They should never be forced to do so. In the most healthy situations, I would expect the church leaders to take an active role in the discipleship of the transgender person attending their church. They should also not be surprised when church members have questions, especially younger children in attendance.

Admittedly, it is the last point that is often a major concern in the church. Many people, understandably, are concerned with how their children will respond. For instance, "Will the presence of a transgender person at the church gatherings lead to confusion for some of the more impressionable people in attendance?" As a pastor and a father, I, too, am concerned with my children and the children in my church being influenced and confused by the world. However, in a situation where church leaders are faithfully teaching God's Word on issues and gender and sexuality, and parents are being equipped to have these difficult but important conversations with their kids, I think that the children will be just fine. I will, however, confess that a church that is not teaching and addressing these topics regularly will be far less equipped and more susceptible to confusion than churches that are equipping members with biblical trust about gender and sexuality. As for the transgender person, I would much rather they attend a church that lovingly challenges their false self-perception than for them to attend one that affirms it.

Churches will require wisdom to produce and teach through various kinds of policies and scenarios. Imagine a scenario when a new student is visiting the church's youth ministry. It is a biological boy who identifies as a girl. How should a church and its leaders address this scenario? If the leaders did not know the new student before the supposed gender transition, then it might be understandable for them to use the preferred gender, name, and pronoun on account of ignorance. Upon awareness of the transition, in time, love should compel us to speak the truth regarding God's will for biological sex and gender. Obviously, the nature of that conversation would depend on whether the student professed to be a believer or an unbeliever. If the student professed to be a believer, then this would be an opportunity for deeper discipleship and a call to repentance in keeping with the faith that they profess. If, however, the student did not profess to be a believer, I believe we should keep the goal of sharing Christ at the top of our priorities. The time will come to address the student's gender confusion in the context of the repentance that accompanies saving faith. Our aim in ministering to lost students is not first and foremost to win them to our side on matters of sexuality and gender, but rather to see them won to Christ. We need not shrink back from speaking the truth in love and kindness, though, nor should we actively accommodate with falsehoods.

THE MAIN THING

We could go on forever with one hypothetical scenario after another, but I would still not be able to exhaust all the possible situations that you will encounter in ministry. So, instead of belaboring the point, I want to conclude with some principles to guide us in loving others well without compromising biblical truth. If you're a pastor or in church leadership, you've got to realize that preparing your congregation begins with you! You cannot wait to have this conversation until it happens because I can assure you it's going to happen. In fact, it's probably already happened in one way or another. We cannot stick our heads in the sand and ignore what is happening around us. The families that God has entrusted to our leadership in the church are already facing these situations. If we are unwilling to address these topics, our people will be unprepared to live faithfully to Christ in an increasingly hostile world. So, pastors, equip your people, form the ministry teams, write the policies with input from wise, mature Christians in your congregation, and ask the Lord to help you.

If we want to know how God's glory is most clearly seen in our words and deeds, we should look to Christ, the image of the invisible God (Col. 1:15). When Christ ministered to sinners, He neither affirmed nor ignored their sin. His ministry aimed to glorify God through the redemption of sinners. His aim was not to reveal sin and then leave people without hope. Jesus revealed sin to draw people to Himself for salvation. Some, like the woman at the well, embraced Jesus. Others, like the rich young ruler, turned away from Jesus. In both cases, Jesus' words were hard but lovingly aimed at redemption. In one case, the words found good soil, and the woman bore fruit in keeping with repentance. In another, the words found no place, and the man turned away because he was in love with something other than God. In ministering to a transgender individual, one must be convinced that faithfulness to Jesus in the ministry of the gospel will ultimately lead to fruitfulness in ministry. This means the same message will bear fruit in some while bearing none in others, and this type of growth is not up to those doing the sowing. It is God who causes such growth.

———

Redemption is what the Christian life is about, isn't it? In most religions, mankind strives to reach God. In Christianity, it is God who reaches out and seeks us. In our final chapter looking at the biblical-theological framework, we'll examine our own place in God's great plans for the world, and where we are in the "already, not yet" equation.

CHAPTER TWELVE

Exploring the Biblical-Theological Framework Five

YOU ARE HERE: Our Place in God's Redemptive Plan

I grew up going to Six Flags Over Texas each summer with my family. Two of my cousins would come spend a week with us and we would go to the local pool and a few parks, but eventually, we would head to Dallas for all the wild rides.

For the first few years, I was too scared to ride anything big, but I overcame my fear (read: "was forced by my sister-in-law") and started riding the roller coasters. Six Flags is sprawling. You can walk and wait for hours! But fortunately, they had misting stations and maps all over the place to take care of you in the sweltering Texas summer heat. On those maps, there was typically an indicator labeled, "You are here."

These indicators oriented guests. It let them know where they were so they could get to where they were going. This could be encouraging or discouraging, depending on where exactly you were located. If you were looking for the parking lot, but you were at the back of the park, it meant you had a long walk. If, however, you were looking for a bathroom and maybe wanted to purchase a $7 Coke, have no fear; these were always near. In this brief chapter, I hope to provide you with something like a "You are here" indicator for where we are in this grand story of Creation, Crisis, Christ, and Creation Regained. Knowing where we are located in God's redemptive plan provides us with a valuable perspective about how to navigate a sexually broken world without losing hope or becoming loveless.

ALREADY, NOT YET

Already. Not yet. You may have heard someone use these words together like this before, but what do they mean? Why are they important? And how can we reconcile these words that seem to be in contradiction to one another? The idea of "already, not yet" describes how we, as Christians, are living in the "in-between" of Christ's first coming and second coming.

One way to illustrate this would be to consider the concept of eternal life. As Christians, we "already" possess eternal life in Christ. Yet, Christians still die. How can this be the case? How can a Christian who possesses eternal life now in the present die? This is where the idea of the "already, not yet" is helpful. Through union with Christ by faith, we are already enjoying some of the benefits of eternal life, like hope, forgiveness, peace, and joy. Yet, there is a day when we will enjoy such benefits in their fullness. So, to say that Christians already possess eternal life yet die does not reveal a contradiction but rather a paradox. The paradox is that while we might die before Christ's second coming, we will certainly be raised to a fully consummated life with God in the new heaven and new earth.

Let's consider some of the Bible's teaching on this idea of the "already, not yet." David Briones mentions five examples of the "already, not yet."[1] He highlights how Scripture speaks of Christians being

- already adopted in Christ (Rom. 8:15), but not yet adopted (Rom. 8:23)
- already redeemed in Christ (Eph. 1:7), but not yet redeemed (Eph. 4:30)
- already sanctified in Christ (1 Cor. 1:2), but not yet sanctified (1 Thess. 5:23–24)
- already saved in Christ (Eph. 2:8), but not yet saved (Rom. 5:9)
- already raised with Christ (Eph. 2:6), but not yet raised (1 Cor. 15:52)

In other words, we are living in a tension, a time in between what God has already accomplished in and through Jesus Christ on our behalf and what God will bring to completion on the day of Christ Jesus. And this is not only true for Christians, but also for the creation, which will fully and finally be regained with Christ's return and His subsequent rule and reign in the new heaven and the new earth. Thus, as Christians now, we look forward to the day when the fullness of our redemption is revealed and enjoyed.

Thinking about our location in the world at this point in redemptive history should temper our expectations in the present and fill us with hope for the future. This concept of the "already, not yet" helps us see where we are at in terms of our location on God's map. We are not fully home yet, but we can be certain that one day we will be.

What this means for us now as we navigate a sexually broken world is that God is with and for His people, regardless of how the world perceives us. As we seek to love others while living faithfully to Christ, we should not be surprised when people do not receive our message of the hope and forgiveness that is offered to sinners in the gospel. Furthermore, the hope of the life to come ought to embolden us to be faithful witnesses to the gospel and not be ashamed of Christ or His gospel (Rom. 1:16).

Why do we need to know where we are at this moment in redemptive history? It is because following Christ can be hard. There is a cost associated with being a disciple of Christ. If we would be faithful followers of Christ, then our ultimate allegiance must be to Him, not our families, our friends, our careers, our political parties, or anything else in this world. Let's face it, that's quite the call on our life as followers of Jesus. But living a life that is informed by this idea of the "already, not yet" strengthens us to see that God has not abandoned His powerful work in our lives. When we face opposition, we should not be surprised. Jesus told us that such opposition would come and is now here. Following Jesus doesn't mean that everyone is going to agree with us, but we need to be very careful not to take such rejection personally. While it may feel personal at times, ultimately those who reject the message of the gospel are rejecting Christ and His genuine offer of salvation to all who would turn away from their sins in repentance and place their trust in Him as their Savior and Lord.

The gospel's message does not originate with us, nor do we have the authority to change it to suit our context better. We are messengers of the gospel, not editors, which is to say that we are tasked with simply delivering His message to others so that they might come to know Him and join us in this tension of living in the "already, not yet."

The truth of the "already, not yet" has profound implications not only for our expectations but also for how we will relate and minister to those who struggle with sexual sin and temptation. At times, when Christ saves a person, they will see the immediate fruit of the Holy Spirit working in their lives. But that fruit might not always manifest itself in the same way in every person.

NOT DEFINED BY STRUGGLE

Let me give you a personal example. I spent the better part of my teenage years in a church with only a few other people my age. To be completely honest, I did not like them. I was the only person in our youth group who went to school outside of the home. I was the only person who played a sport. I was the only person who was allowed to have a girlfriend. I enjoyed secular music and watched PG-13 movies. I didn't feel like I had anything in common with anyone in my church, but I had to go because my older brother was the pastor. Most Sundays, I would run the sound system in the back of the auditorium and sleep during the sermon. I wore my oversized Starter jacket to give me cover, but the red mark on my forehead after every service was a dead giveaway. The pastor's little brother was a heathen.

There are almost certainly sins in our lives that we will continue to wage war against until the day that Jesus returns.

But something radically changed when God saved me at age seventeen. I went from having nothing in common with the other students in my youth group to feeling like they were my family. I moved from not liking them to truly loving them. Many of these guys in my youth group would go on to become dear friends, even groomsmen in my wedding. This change was nearly instantaneous with my conversion to Christ. When Christ saved me, it was as if I was immediately granted new eyes to see these people as brothers and sisters in Christ. God mercifully delivered me from this obvious example of sin and drew me into a deeper fellowship with Himself and other believers in my church. I still feel this to this day. That is not to say that I am still very close to all of the people—we all grew up, got married, had kids, started careers, moved away from home, etc.—but I have the conviction that I will always have greater commonality and fellowship with my brothers and sisters in Christ than I will with unbelievers who share the same taste in music or cheer for the same sports teams. Some things in my life radically changed when Christ saved me.

I'm sure you have either heard this or experienced it as well. Just recall how many testimonies you have heard of people who were addicted to alcohol, drugs, or pornography before their conversion, but almost immediately upon trusting Christ, their desire for these sinful vices disappeared. Sometimes this happens, and we give God all the glory for such testimonies.

Yet, while some sins may seem conquered to the point of almost disappearing at the time of our conversion, there are almost certainly other sins in our lives that we will continue to wage war against until the day that Jesus returns.

Want to know one of the sins I have noticed that I must continually war against? It is the sin of worry. If worry were an Olympic sport, I would be dangerously close to capturing the gold medal. Now, at this point, some of you may want to counsel me, and tell me that it is "normal to worry," but, if that is the case, let me pull back the curtain a little more for you. At the heart of my struggle with the sin of worry is a lack of trust in God's sovereign rule over my life and the life of my family. When I say I struggle with the sin of worry, I'm not talking about something like "I'm worried we are going to be late to the baseball game." I mean, I worry that God's plan for my family and me might not be good. While I have read the wisdom literature of the book of Proverbs, I've also read the book of Job. A righteous life does not guarantee you an easy or prosperous life. I know that I can be faithful to Christ and be struck with cancer. These are not in contradiction with one another.

I know that "all things are working together for my good" as someone who loves Christ and has been called according to His purpose, but that passage does not mean that everything I experience in this life is good in and of itself. Cancer is not good. Car wrecks are not good. The stroke that killed my father was not good. Yet, Christ is still good and intends good for me, even when bad things are present in my life. I'm intellectually aware of this truth, yet I have to fight to believe it. I have prayed and pleaded with the Lord to deliver me from this worry. I know that it is not His revealed will for my life. Yet, here I am, still struggling with it. Maybe one day I will have victory over it, but for now, it is a battle. I must seek to put to death the fleshly, sinful impulse to doubt the goodness of God and worry about my future, which is ultimately in His hands.

I should not regard myself as a "worrying Christian," as if this is my lot in life and there is no hope of full and final deliverance.

What does this have to do with the "already, not yet"? Everything. While some sins, as was true in my experience, may cease to be the primary battleground for your sanctification after your conversion, there may be other "besetting sins" that you must continue to deal with and address until the time when the work of our redemption that has "already" begun is fully realized at Christ's return. We need this category of the "already, not yet" if we are going to fight our own sins well while helping others to do the same. We should not let our present struggle with sin define who we are in Christ. I should not regard myself as a "worrying Christian," as if this is my lot in life and there is no hope of full and final deliverance. Furthermore, I should not attempt to redefine my worry as something acceptable to God. Instead, I should fight the battle against the sin of worry in the present, considering the future victory that is guaranteed for me in Christ. The certainty of this victory over my sin and your sin in the future (the "not yet") ought to empower us to fight against this sin in the present because of what Christ has "already" accomplished.

But there is more benefit to this idea of the "already, not yet" than just our own personal battles with sin. The concept of the "already, not yet" ought to remind us that just as we are works in process by God's grace, our fellow brothers and sisters in Christ are also in process. We call this idea of being a "work in process" by God's grace the work of progressive sanctification. To be sure, the Scriptures certainly teach an "already" aspect of our sanctification, but that is not in contradiction to the "not yet" of our sanctification. God has so orchestrated our lives as believers that He continually works in us through the Holy Spirit so we may be "conformed to the image of his Son" (Rom. 8:29). So, even as we work out our own salvation in "fear and trembling" (Phil. 2:12), we need to be mindful that every true Christian is on this same journey. Being mindful of this process should not only strengthen our own resolve to follow Christ but also lead us to encourage others to keep growing in their conformity to Christ and help us be patient with others, just as God is so patient with us.

We've covered a lot of ground in this book. I do hope that as you have read and studied these topics and seek to apply them in your own life that you will wield the truth of God's Word like a surgeon's scalpel instead of a bludgeoning hammer. The point is not to win an argument. The point is to be faithful to the call that God has given us as faithful followers of Christ. To be sure, at times, the scalpel will inflict pain. It will cut deep. Scripture makes no promise that God's truth will not be offensive. Yet, a scalpel aims to heal and make whole what is broken and diseased.

Remember why we are studying these things: to love our LGBTQ friends and family well without compromising the biblical truth that God intends to use to save them from their sins, just as He did and does with you and with me.

CHAPTER THIRTEEN

Birthdays and Bathrooms— Living as Christians in Public

Imagine that your daughter is invited to a classmate's birthday party. You read the invitation and notice that it is from a parent that you have known casually through your daughter's school for a few years, but you do not recognize the name of the classmate on the invitation. "Sam," you say out loud. "I don't think I know Sam."

Your daughter overhears your confusion and explains that her friend Samantha now goes by Sam. As you reread the birthday invitation, you notice the use of male pronouns in reference to Sam and the request from Sam's parents to purchase toys and clothing that would stereotypically be for a male child. You ask your daughter for clarification and learn that her friend Samantha/Sam believes she is now a "he." Sam is in the midst of a social transition, which, in this case, entails not only a name change but also some nonpermanent outward appearance changes in an attempt to conform to their newly perceived gender.

What do you do as a parent in this type of situation? Do you honor the parents' wishes and buy the gifts they request for Sam? Do you allow your child to continue to be friends with Sam? Does she go to the party? How do we navigate these types of public situations with both love and truth?

Or here's another scenario. Let's say that you are a church leader, and a member of your church comes up to ask you about a situation he is facing at work. His company has just passed a new email signature policy requiring all employees to include their preferred pronouns. The church member feels uncomfortable with this new policy because he feels like it forces him to affirm a specific ideology that is contrary to his understanding of biblical gender and sexuality. At the same time, he's the breadwinner to a family of four children. He's worried that if he does not conform to the new policy, he will lose his job and the family will suffer. How do you counsel this concerned church member?

These scenarios are all too real. The difficulty of navigating the public square as a Christian gets more challenging with each day that passes. And I have no reason to believe that this is going to change any time soon. This reality, however, should not leave us in despair. As Christians, God has revealed His will for our lives in His Word. Now, I know that Scripture does not explicitly address the two scenarios we've just pondered, but it does provide us with sufficient wisdom and direction for navigating difficult situations. Below, I hope to demonstrate how we might lean on God's Word to guide us through the public square with love and truth.

PARENTING IN THE PUBLIC SQUARE

In the first scenario I posed above, we concluded by considering a few questions that arise in social relationships with others in the public square who do not share our Christian understanding of gender and sexuality. In some ways, the principles we have covered in other chapters also apply here. For instance, parents have a biblical responsibility to protect their children not only from physical harm but also from spiritual harm. So, again, it is entirely appropriate and right for a parent to wrestle with whether they want to allow their child to continue to have a friendship with a particular child or to attend a particular school. A parent should not feel shame about wrestling with these types of situations. Their God-given responsibility is to raise their child in the "training and instruction of the Lord" (Eph. 6:4). Parents, don't shy away from this responsibility because you are worried that someone might not like you or your children.

What does it look like to raise your child in the "training and instruction of the Lord"? I believe Deuteronomy 6 provides a tremendous guide for us. So, let's take a deeper look at this important passage. Here we see Moses use repetition and summary to drive home the importance of the laws that he just taught the people in Deuteronomy 5. In terms of repetition, Moses tells the people again that these "commands, decrees, and laws" from the Lord were given to the Israelites to teach them how to live in the promised land. As the people obeyed, they would enjoy God's blessing in the land.

These instructions were for the Israelites, their children, and their grandchildren, which is another way to say each generation of Israelites needed to know and obey these commands that the Lord gave His people. The idea in the passage is not that just these three generations would need to hear these things, but that each successive generation of God's people would need to hear them.

Another way of putting this would be to say that you and the next generation should be taught to know and obey the commands of the Lord. The Israelites had a divine obligation to know and obey for themselves, but also to make sure that the next generation of Israelites knew and obeyed the commands of the Lord. So, part of obedience to the command was to make sure that children and grandchildren in the community knew and obeyed the commands of the Lord. If only the present generation were the focus, then the people were disobeying God's command. So, we as parents obey God as we instruct our children to obey God.

After repeating the need for the people to obey the law of the Lord, Moses moves to a summary of the law. As one Old Testament scholar, Peter Craigie, put it, Deuteronomy 6:4–5 is the "principal law" or "main law" of the Israelites. He writes,

> The command to love is central because the whole book is concerned with the renewing of the covenant with God, and although the renewal demanded obedience, that obedience would be possible only when it was a response of love to the God who had brought the people out of Egypt and was leading them into the promised land.[1]

As the principal law, our passage commands God's people to love Him with all their being.

Let's take a little closer look at verses 4–5.

First, we note that the passage begins with a declaration about God: "Hear, O Israel: The LORD our God, the LORD is one." These words are known as the *Shema*, which is a Jewish confession about the Lord. In Hebrew, the first word in the phrase is "shema," which means "listen or hear." The whole phrase sounds something like this: "Shema, Yisrael, YHWH (Adonai) Eloheinu, YHWH (Adonai) echad." The Jews would repeat this confession in prayer daily.

Eventually, within Judaism, other passages of Scripture were added to this confession (Deut. 11:13–21; Num. 15:37–41). This confession was a pronouncement of absolute allegiance to the Lord alone. As the first two commandments of the Ten Commandments told the people, they were to have no other gods before the Lord, and they were not to make "an image" to represent the Lord. Taken together with the first two commandments, we can conclude that Deuteronomy 6:4 is an expression of monotheism, which is the belief that there is only one true God.

This passage does not deny that the other nations had their own gods that they worshiped. Furthermore, this passage does not deny that the so-called gods of the other nations were likely demonic, meaning that demonic activity was associated with the worship of these so-called other gods. Such demonic activity likely caused the people to be deceived into thinking that they were actual, self-sufficient gods. It is reasonable to believe that surrounding nations were deceived and manipulated by spiritual beings, demons that would manifest themselves in and through the idols that the people had fashioned from metal and wood. Deuteronomy 6:4 is not denying that such events happened. Instead, Deuteronomy 6:4 is saying that while at times it might appear that there are other gods like our God, they are not really gods. They are not worthy of the title "God." For the Israelites, there was only one God, Creator and Sustainer of all things, to whom they were to be loyal. And, when compared to the Lord, all of the gods of the nations were no gods at all.

So, here in verse 4, we have a declaration of the Lord as the unique, supreme God over all. This is Israel's God. This is the God to whom they owe their full allegiance. This is the God that no other being in the universe can challenge. This is the God beyond all comparison. And this God, the Lord, commands that His people, who He redeemed from Egypt, are to love Him with the entirety of their being, which is the point of verse 5. "Love the LORD your God with all your heart and with all your soul and with all your strength." The point here is not so much that we need to separate the heart, soul, and strength and figure out how to love with each of these different aspects of our being. Instead, the "heart, soul, and strength" are representative of the whole person. There is not a single aspect of our being that is not claimed by the Lord. He is worthy of *all* our love with *all* our life.

> There is not a single aspect of our being that is not claimed by the Lord. He is worthy of all our love with all our life.

The question that comes, then, is: How does someone grow in loving the Lord with the entirety of their being? In other words, how do we as parents both grow in our love for the Lord and teach our children to do so as well? Verses 6–9 tell us. This life of full-fledged love of the Lord requires that the commands of the Lord take root in us through meditation on His law. One thinks of Psalm 1, which speaks of meditating on the law of the Lord "day and night." In verses 6–9, we see that during day and night and in every place, God's people should think of His law.

If God's people are going to keep God's commands, then our lives must be marked by meditation on the Word of the Lord. If our hearts want to grow in love for the Lord, then we must know and obey His Word. If we desire for our children to know these truths,

then we will encourage and provide opportunities for them as well.
But what is this relationship between meditating on God's law
and growing in our love for God? Well, it is based on this principle:
What we meditate on, think about, memorize, and fixate on impacts
how we live and think in the world as the people of God. God has
designed us this way. We become like the things that we meditate on.
You may say, "What do you mean by that? What do you mean that
we become like the things that we meditate on?" Essentially, what I
mean is what Psalm 115:1–8 says about idolatry. Listen to what the
psalmist writes,

> Not to us, LORD, not to us
> > but to your name be the glory,
> > because of your love and faithfulness.
> Why do the nations say,
> > "Where is their God?"
> Our God is in heaven;
> > he does whatever pleases him.
> But their idols are silver and gold,
> > made by human hands.
> They have mouths, but cannot speak,
> > eyes, but cannot see.
> They have ears, but cannot hear,
> > noses, but cannot smell.
> They have hands, but cannot feel,
> > feet, but cannot walk,
> > nor can they utter a sound with their throats.
> Those who make them will be like them,
> > and so will all who trust in them.

Those who make idols and trust in idols will become like those idols. But you say, "That passage doesn't say anything about meditation. You said we become like the things that we meditate on. Where is that in the text?" Good question. Meditation on the Lord and His law is what He has prescribed to keep us from the sin of idolatry. As Moses told the people, "These commandments that I give you today are to be on your hearts. Impress them on your children. Talk about them when you sit at home and when you walk along the road, when you lie down and when you get up. Tie them as symbols on your hands and bind them on your foreheads. Write them on the doorframes of your houses and on your gates" (Deut. 6:6–9).

In other words, do whatever it takes to get these truths into you and in your children. Meditate on them. Think deeply about them. Make them a matter of the heart, that you might not simply know these things but cherish them. Why? Because God desires our hearts to be turned to Him! God is not interested in our ceremonies. He is interested in our affection. He desires for us to love Him, and He has designated that we demonstrate our love for Him by trusting Him enough to obey what He commands. This requires us to believe that God's will for us is better than our own.

So, we show our love for God by trusting Him enough to obey what He has said, even when it conflicts with the values of the society that we live in. We hold fast to the belief that there is only one true God, the Lord, who has revealed Himself in Jesus Christ for our salvation, even while the world says that there are multiple ways to God. We hold fast to the belief that God is the Creator and Sustainer of all life and that when He created humanity, He made humanity in His image and designated them male and female. We have a responsibility to not only believe this but to teach this to our children as well.

We fulfill the law of loving God and others when we, with the entirety of our being, trust and obey when God commands us to honor our parents, not murder or hate others, not commit sexual sins, not lie or steal or covet our neighbor, even while the world that we live in says otherwise. And when we obey the Lord instead of the world, we are demonstrating that our allegiance is ultimately to Him, and that we love Him more than being accepted by those who do not love Him.

Herein lies the relationship between love and law. Obeying God rather than others shows that we trust Him more than others and that we desire to glorify Him more than others, which shows that He is our treasure, He is who we value more than anything else. And if we are going to grow in this love, then we must meditate on the Lord and His perfect law of liberty in Christ to us. This is how we grow to love the one true God in Spirit and in truth with all our heart, soul, mind, and strength, as Jesus would put it in Luke 10:27. God longs for us to love Him and demonstrate such love for Him by trusting Him, by believing in Him enough to obey Him. And impressing this upon our children is how we raise children in the "training and instruction of the Lord."

Does this guarantee that all our children will come to faith in Christ? No. Salvation belongs to the Lord, not parents (Jonah 2:9). Yet, our sovereign God is a God of means who often chooses to use faithful parents as instruments of His saving grace in the lives of their children and grandchildren. Furthermore, God is often pleased to use parents to equip their children to think biblically about matters like gender and sexuality. As parents, will you do this perfectly? No. Do you need God's grace as much as your children? Yes. Am I stressing these things because I want to put pressure on you? Not at all. I'm sure you already feel plenty of pressure as a parent. But I am stressing these things because they are important. If we are not careful, we can become so overwhelmed by the near-constant changes and demands that we encounter in society that we forget or neglect the more important, unchanging matters in life.

We must seek to cultivate a vision of faith in and obedience to God that will serve generations of Christians who will continue to wrestle with difficult questions like these and those we are yet even to imagine.

What does all of this have to do with those questions we asked about the birthday party at the beginning of the chapter? All this talk about the spiritual formation of our children through meditation and instruction is both the foundation and the context in which we must wrestle with these kinds of questions. It will not be enough to simply say, "Don't go to the party," or "Just buy them a gift card," or "Pull your kids out of public school," or "Get involved with the local school board and make a change," or "Find a Christian school in your area," or "Have a conversation with the classmates' parents," or any other host of legitimate responses to those questions. What we need in these situations is a biblical-theological framework from which we not only view the world but also our role in the world as parents. We must seek to cultivate a vision of faith in and obedience to God that will serve generations of Christians who will continue to wrestle with difficult questions like these and those we are yet even to imagine.

In summary, we must be okay with being different in society. I'm not advocating for Christians to be needlessly weird. You don't have to learn how to sew or churn your own butter to be faithful to Jesus.

But we do need to accept the cost of following Jesus and teach our children that Jesus is worth it! And this leads me to the next scenario we posed at the beginning.

TRUSTING JESUS IN THE PUBLIC SQUARE

It is crucial that we learn how to follow Jesus, even when it seems to cost us everything. And who better to listen to than Jesus Himself! In Matthew 10, Jesus exhorts His disciples to place their trust wholly in Him as they obey His call on their lives. Simply put, following Jesus will come with a cost, but that cost should not deter our obedience to Him. According to Jesus, "You will be hated by everyone because of me, but the one who stand firm to the end will be saved" (v. 22). Jesus' call on our life is not to prosperity or popularity but perseverance in the face of adversity. Yet, what compels us to persevere is the promise that He will take care of us. While we may be hated "by everyone," we can rest assured that we are loved by God (vv. 29–31).

What this means for how we navigate issues—like losing our job because of our refusal to comply with speech policies that violate not only our religious liberty but also contradict our biblical convictions about gender and sexuality—is that we can trust God with our obedience to Him. We do not have to, nor should we equivocate on obeying God rather than others.

If God's Word is clear on a matter, then we can trust that He will take care of us and our family as we seek to conform and submit to His revealed will in Scripture. We cannot love our careers or our sense of security more than we love God. To do so would be idolatry, something that Scripture explicitly and repeatedly prohibits. So, whether it's a decision about a birthday party or a boardroom, we are called to trust God who has demonstrated His love for us in Jesus Christ. We can trust Him! We *must* trust Him. He is faithful. He will take care of His people. He will take care of you.

"And Such Were Some of You"— The Power of the Gospel of Christ

I will never forget preaching the Sunday after the Supreme Court decided to legalize same-sex marriage. People were dejected. They were fearful. They were wondering what was going to happen to the United States. Would pastors and churches be required to perform same-sex weddings? Would Christians be imprisoned for saying that same-sex marriage was sinful? What would happen to Christian business owners who refused to use their creative gifts and expressions to celebrate same-sex marriages?

I do not have the space to address all such questions here. In this concluding chapter, I want to address the underlying fear and despair I saw within my congregation and among many other professing Christians. Why? Because I am still sensing it and seeing it today regarding the topics that we have considered in this book. And just as I did on that summer morning back in 2015, I want to close by providing a few reflections on how I believe we should respond not with fear and despair but with conviction, clarity, and confidence because of Christ Jesus!

In 1 Corinthians 6:9–11, the apostle Paul wrote, "Or do you not know that wrongdoers will not inherit the kingdom of God? Do not be deceived: Neither the sexually immoral nor idolaters nor adulterers nor men who have sex with men nor thieves nor the greedy nor drunkards nor slanderers nor swindlers will inherit the kingdom of God. And that is what some of you were. But you were washed, you were sanctified, you were justified in the name of the Lord Jesus Christ and by the Spirit of our God." I believe this passage points us in the right direction for how we should respond to our present societal moment.

First, I believe this passage demonstrates that we should respond to our present societal moment with gospel conviction. As Paul asked the Corinthian church, so he is asking us if we know that "wrongdoers will not inherit the kingdom of God." In brief, God's kingdom refers to the eternal life or resurrection mentioned by Paul in 1 Corinthians 15:50, where he states, "flesh and blood cannot inherit the kingdom of God." Only those with a transformed life will inherit the resurrection, which entails the new heaven and the new earth with the new Jerusalem and God's presence for all eternity, which we considered in chapter 9. Do you know this? Do you realize that eternity is at stake?

Do we believe this or not? Do we agree with what God's Word teaches here? I would go so far as to ask you to ask God to haunt your soul with this gospel conviction that "wrongdoers will not inherit God's kingdom." Why? Because if you do not believe in the reality of sin, death, and hell, you will live and die in apathy toward the eternal destiny of your neighbors, your children, and your enemies. Paul wanted the Corinthians and us to have gospel conviction about eternity! God's inheritance is only for God's children. Those who have been born again. Those who have been declared righteous by faith in Jesus Christ! If we are not convinced that heaven and hell hang in the balance, we will not be a people of gospel conviction. Instead, we will merely be a people of gospel convenience.

So, what is the gospel that we must have great conviction about? This leads to our second response to our present societal moment. We must respond with gospel clarity. God's Word does not leave us in the dark regarding the gospel and its expectation. God calls us to repent (turn continually from sin) and trust that Jesus Christ has suffered the punishment for our sin and given us the eternal life due for His righteous life. And the gospel does not leave us guessing about the things that we are to repent of. It makes it clear what is considered rebellion against God (Gal. 5:19–21; Eph. 5:5; Rev. 22:15).

Paul makes this clear in 1 Corinthians 6:10, where he mentions a vice list. What is he doing with this list? New Testament scholar Anthony Thiselton explains,

He is not describing the qualifications required for an entrance examination; he is comparing habituated actions, which by definition can find no place in God's reign for the welfare of all, with those qualities in accordance with which Christian believers need to be transformed if they belong authentically to God's new creation in Christ. Everything which persistently opposes what it is to be Christlike must undergo change if those who practice such things wish to call themselves Christians and to look forward to resurrection with Christ.[1]

In other words, Paul is saying, "One cannot claim to follow Christ and yet perpetually live in rebellion against Christ." One cannot claim to honor Christ while honoring idols. One cannot claim to love Christ while lusting after people and things that Christ has forbidden. Who then will inherit the kingdom of God? New Testament scholars Roy Ciampa and Brian Rosner answer, writing, "The answer is, those whose faith commitment to Christ leads them to reject the immoral, greedy, and idolatrous behavior which marks the lives of pagans."[2]

The kingdom of God is for those who have responded to the message of the kingdom: "Turn from your sin and believe in the gospel!" Those who have not repented in submission to the lordship of Christ have not truly believed the gospel and been saved. They will not inherit the kingdom of God! The kingdom of God is reserved for those who have loved Christ more than their desires, be those sexual, religious, material, or social!

We must maintain this type of gospel clarity in response to the challenges that we face in society. The answer to the challenges that we are facing is not to relabel and repackage sin as something that is acceptable or "no big deal" to God. The answer is to be clear about our sinful condition and God's remedy through Christ! And oh, how great a remedy it is, which leads to a final response.

We must respond to our present societal moment with gospel confidence! Or, another way to state this would be to say we must respond with gospel hope. As I have reflected upon much of the public conversation that has taken place on these topics of gender and sexuality, I have witnessed a lot of lamenting. I am not saying that there is no place for lament and sorrow, but what I am saying is that we need more than lament and sorrow. We need hope! Confidence in the power of the gospel of Christ!

We cannot simply read 1 Corinthians 6:9–10 and not read verse 11, which says, "And that is what some of you were. But you were washed, you were sanctified, you were justified in the name of the Lord Jesus Christ and by the Spirit of our God." Paul had confidence in the power of the gospel to transform people. Yet, I fear that, at times, Christians get so caught up in the "sinfulness of sin" that they forget the power of the gospel of Jesus Christ. As I scroll through social media, I sometimes get the feeling that people know something that I don't know, like maybe someone had found Jesus' bones in a tomb in Jerusalem or that someone had definitively proven that the Scriptures were false. But that is never the case. Instead, it seems that people are just surprised to find that humanity is sinful, and somehow that sinfulness has trumped the power of God to save and transform people.

Sure, the types of things that we are seeing in our society might feel like rather new expressions of sinful rebellion against God, but rebellion against God is not new. We must remember that first-century Christianity thrived in a context where sexual immorality was prevalent. And yet, the Roman Empire has fallen, while the church of Christ still stands!

How does this happen? Well, it's pretty obvious from verse 11. As Christ through the gospel invades these pagan places, lives are radically transformed. Note the passive voice of the verbs in verse 11: You were washed, you were sanctified, you were justified. The people of the early church did not change their own lives—they didn't clean themselves up. They did not set themselves apart. They did not make themselves righteous before God. No way! These people were spiritually dead in trespasses and sins (Eph. 2:1). They were powerless, sinners and enemies of God (Rom. 5).

So what happened? According to Acts 18, God commanded Paul

in a vision to "keep on speaking, do not be silent" about Christ in Corinth because the Lord had "many people in the city." God promised Paul that He would be with him as he preached and persuaded, and according to verse 8, "Many of the Corinthians, who heard Paul believed and were baptized" (see vv. 8–10). As God empowered Paul's preaching, many heard the gospel and were saved. They were transformed!

We can have confidence in the gospel because of the God of the gospel. He accompanies the preaching of the gospel and brings about spiritual life through the supernatural work of the Holy Spirit! The message that we believe and that we proclaim, the gospel of Jesus Christ, specializes in taking the sexually immoral, the idolater, the homosexual, the thief, the greedy person, the drunk, the reviler, and the swindler, and making them into citizens of the kingdom of God who have been washed, who have been sanctified, who have been justified "in the name of the Lord Jesus Christ and by the Spirit of our God" (1 Cor. 6:11).

This is no time to lose hope. If God can save you and me, He can save anyone. This is no time to put aside the command of Christ to love God and neighbor out of despair. This is a time to be faithful to God as disciples of Jesus Christ who are empowered by the Holy Spirit and known for love without compromising the truth that sets people free. John 8:31–32 tells us:

Jesus said, "If you hold to my teaching, you are really my disciples. Then you will know the truth, and the truth will set you free."

Acknowledgments

I would be remiss to not thank those who have supported and encouraged me along the way. First, I am grateful to God for the churches that He has allowed me to serve over the past seventeen years of ministry. They have consistently demonstrated a loving patience toward me when I was not always known for love in my preaching and teaching. Second, I would thank God for my friends who have served as a constant sounding board and source of encouragement and correction. In particular, I think of Eric Nimtz, Stephen Partain, Andrew Walker, Josh Wester, Dustin Bruce, Erik Reed, Dean Inserra, Daniel Darling, and Cory Barnes. To be sure, their inclusion here should not be construed to mean that they would agree with me at every point in this book. They are their own men. Yet, in various ways over the course of this project, they have helped me along the way, and for that, I am grateful. I would also like to thank my literary agent, Brad Byrd, with Wadestone Inc., for his persistent help and representation during this process. Furthermore, I am grateful to Drew Dyck and the team at Moody

Publishers for their work and support of this book. Thank you for this opportunity.

Finally, I would like to thank my family, especially my wife, Hannah, for giving me the encouragement and time to write. Apart from my salvation in Christ, my wife is God's greatest gift to me. To my kids, Carter, Jude, Weston, Eden, and Willow, thank you for being a welcomed distraction from the seriousness of this sort of book. I love each of you so much! I pray that this book will help you and your future families as you attempt to live as followers of Jesus, who are known for love.

Last, I want to dedicate this book to my mother, Kay. If I ever met someone who embodied a "love that rejoices in truth," it is my mother. I have watched her weep over her family and friends whom she loves deeply in the truth. If a relative who didn't know Jesus was ever nearing death, my mother wanted to be there to plead with them to put their trust in Jesus. She wants everyone to know and love the Savior she has grown to know and love over all these decades of faith. I cannot recall a day when I lived at home when I didn't wake to find her at the kitchen table reading her Bible with both elbows planted firmly on each side while praying for her family and friends. Thank you for setting such a wonderful example, Mom. I am grateful to God that you are my mother!

Notes

CHAPTER 1: CREATION: "AND IT WAS VERY GOOD"

1. Sandra L. Richter, *Stewards of Eden: What Scripture Says About the Environment and Why It Matters* (Downers Grove, IL: IVP Academic, 2020), 7.
2. John H. Walton, *Ancient Near Eastern Thought and the Old Testament: Introducing the Conceptual World of the Hebrew Bible*, 2nd ed. (Grand Rapids, MI: Baker Academic, 2018), 158.
3. Richter, *Stewards of Eden*, 7–8.
4. "This is Adam, the collective Hebrew term for 'humanity.' This creature, unlike all the others, is made in the very *image* of God." Sandra L. Richter, *The Epic of Eden: A Christian Entry into the Old Testament* (Downers Grove, IL: IVP Academic, 2008), 102.
5. John H. Walton, *The Lost World of Genesis One: Ancient Cosmology and the Origins Debate* (Downers Grove, IL: IVP Academic, 2009), 148.
6. Richard Lints, *Identity and Idolatry: The Image of God and Its Inversion* (Downers Grove, IL: IVP Academic, 2015), 32.
7. Richter, *The Epic of Eden*, 92.
8. Herman Bavinck, *Reformed Dogmatics*, vol. 2: *God and Creation*, ed. John Bolt, trans. John Vriend (Grand Rapids, MI: Baker Academic, 2003), 407.
9. As D. A. Carson summarizes Francis Schaeffer's important interpretive question regarding Genesis 1–11, "What is the least that Genesis 1–11 must be saying in order for the book of Genesis, and the rest of the Bible, to be coherent and true?" D. A. Carson, "The Many Facets of the Current Discussion," in *The*

Enduring Authority of the Christian Scriptures (Grand Rapids, MI: Eerdmans, 2016), 36.

10. "In our circumstances, we are not helped by the familiar debates over 'creation.' It does not help us make our way through this world and the urgent issues of our times to know how long ago 'this world' was made. Or how long God took to make it. Or precisely what means God used to bring the world into being. These questions may be fascinating puzzles for some people, but answers to them do not constitute a doctrine of creation that articulates our convictions about God's world, who this God is, how we find life, and the purpose of creation that teaches us the way of life." Jonathan R. Wilson, *God's Good World: Reclaiming the Doctrine of Creation* (Grand Rapids, MI: Baker Academic, 2013), vii.

11. The material that follows draws heavily upon the words, ideas, and insight of Iain Provan, found in Iain W. Provan, *Seeking What Is Right: The Old Testament and the Good Life* (Waco, TX: Baylor University Press, 2020), 4–15.

12. Provan, *Seeking What Is Right*, 4.

13. Ibid.

14. Michael F. Bird, *Evangelical Theology: A Biblical and Systematic Introduction*, 2nd ed. (Grand Rapids, MI: Zondervan Academic, 2020), 228.

15. Ibid.

16. The preceding sentences depend heavily on the description from Michael Bird in *Evangelical Theology*, 228.

CHAPTER 2: CRISIS: NOT THE WAY IT'S SUPPOSED TO BE

1. I'm grateful to Cornelius Plantinga for this description of life in a fallen world. Cornelius Plantinga Jr., *Not the Way It's Supposed to Be: A Breviary of Sin* (Grand Rapids, MI: Eerdmans, 1995).

2. "The concept of sin makes no sense if human life, taken as a whole, is purposeless—only 'the outcome of accidental collocations of atoms,' as Bertrand Russell once put it—for, at its core, human sin is a violation of our human *end*, which is to build shalom and thus to glorify and enjoy God forever." Plantinga Jr., *Not the Way It's Supposed to Be*, 17.

3. For an example of this argument, see Gregory K. Beale, *The Temple and the Church's Mission: A Biblical Theology of the Dwelling Place of God* (Downers Grove, IL: IVP Academic, 2005).

4. Herman Bavinck, *Reformed Dogmatics*, vol. 3: *Sin and Salvation in Christ*, ed. John Bolt, trans. John Vriend (Grand Rapids, MI: Baker Academic, 2003), 31.

5. Thomas H. McCall, *Against God and Nature: The Doctrine of Sin*, Foundations of Evangelical Theology Series (Wheaton, IL: Crossway, 2019), 21.

6. Ibid.
7. Ibid.
8. Anna Brown, "More than Twice as Many Americans Support than Oppose the #MeToo Movement," *Pew Research Center's Social & Demographic Trends Project*, September 29, 2022, https://www.pewresearch.org/social-trends/2022/09/29/more-than-twice-as-many-americans-support-than-oppose-the-metoo-movement/.

CHAPTER 3: IS HOMOSEXUALITY REALLY IN THE BIBLE?

1. See D. A. Carson, *The Gospel According to John*, The Pillar New Testament Commentary (Grand Rapids, MI: Eerdmans, 1991), 488–89.
2. Raymond E. Brown, ed., *The Epistles of John*, The Anchor Bible, vol. 30 (Garden City, NY: Doubleday, 1982), 619.
3. An example of this can be seen in the New International Version (2011) in 1 Corinthians 6:9.
4. "Sexual Orientation and Gender Diversity," American Psychological Association, https://www.apa.org/topics/lgbtq. I found this definition prior to reading Preston Sprinkle's book (cited below), but given that Sprinkle opens his chapter entitled "The Biblical Writers Didn't Know About Sexual Orientation" with the APA's definition of sexual orientation, and that I will be drawing heavily from his book, I wanted to add this clarifying comment.
5. David P. Gushee and Glen Harold Stassen, *Kingdom Ethics: Following Jesus in Contemporary Context*, 2nd ed. (Grand Rapids, MI: Eerdmans, 2016), 265.
6. Robert A. J. Gagnon, ed., *The Bible and Homosexual Practice: Texts and Hermeneutics* (Nashville, TN: Abingdon Press, 2011), 380.
7. "For Paul, homosexuality was simply a further extreme of the corruption inherent in sexual passion itself. It did not spring from a different kind of desire, but simply from desire itself." Dale B. Martin, *Sex and the Single Savior: Gender and Sexuality in Biblical Interpretation* (Louisville, KY: Westminster John Knox Press, 2006), 59.
8. Coupled with this argument regarding "nature" is often the idea that what Paul was dealing with here were "non-procreative" sexual acts, and thus primarily about retaining gender hierarchy from the ancient world.
9. Colby Martin, *Unclobber: Rethinking Our Misuse of the Bible on Homosexuality*, expanded edition with study guide (Louisville, KY: Westminster John Knox Press, 2022), 127–35.
10. For an example of this type of argument, see John Boswell, *Christianity, Social Tolerance, and Homosexuality: Gay People in Western Europe from the*

Beginning of the Christian Era to the Fourteenth Century (Chicago, IL: University of Chicago Press, 1980).

11. David P. Gushee, *Changing Our Mind: Definitive 3rd Edition of the Landmark Call for Inclusion of LGBTQ Christians with Response to Critics* (Canton, MI: Read the Spirit Books, 2017), 9.

12. Matthew Vines, *God and the Gay Christian: The Biblical Case in Support of Same-Sex Relationships* (New York, NY: Convergent Books, 2015), 39–40.

13. Bernadette J. Brooten, *Love Between Women: Early Christian Responses to Female Homoeroticism*, The Chicago Series on Sexuality, History, and Society (Chicago, IL: University of Chicago Press, 1996).

14. Preston Sprinkle, *Does the Bible Support Same-Sex Marriage?: 21 Conversations from a Historically Christian View* (Colorado Springs, CO: David C Cook, 2023), 112. To be fair to Sprinkle, in the paragraph above this summary, he writes, "Again, I'm not saying these authors believed in the same thing that we call same-sex orientation. But there is at least some overlap, some semblance of our modern concept. Sexual behavior is described as the by-product of an innate desire." I want to mention this because I am drawing upon Sprinkle's helpful summary of Brooten's work, not to suggest that he would fully agree with my conclusions in this chapter.

15. Brooten, *Love Between Women*, 361.

16. I am drawing upon Sprinkle's use of the terms "some semblance, some overlap" here. I'm not suggesting that he is or would make the same argument regarding the use of terms and categories. Sprinkle, *Does the Bible Support Same-Sex Marriage?*, 112.

17. For examples of different scholars who see Paul as drawing from Leviticus, see Anthony C. Thiselton, *The First Epistle to the Corinthians: A Commentary on the Greek Text*, New International Greek Testament Commentary (Grand Rapids, MI: Eerdmans, 2000), 440–53.

18. Gordon J. Wenham, *The Book of Leviticus*, The New International Commentary on the Old Testament (Grand Rapids, MI: Eerdmans, 1979), 259.

19. We will consider more about the Old Testament context in the next chapter when we look at Jesus' teaching on marriage and the implications that has for understanding what His disposition would have been toward homosexuality.

20. Sprinkle points out this same example. See Sprinkle, *Does the Bible Support Same-Sex Marriage?*, 132.

21. Brooten, *Love Between Women*, 244, as quoted in Kevin DeYoung, *What Does the Bible Really Teach About Homosexuality?* (Wheaton, IL: Crossway, 2015), 84–85.

22. Louis Crompton, *Homosexuality & Civilization* (Cambridge, MA: The Belknap Press of Harvard Univ. Press, 2006), 114, as quoted in Kevin DeYoung, *What Does the Bible Really Teach About Homosexuality?* (Wheaton, IL: Crossway, 2015), 86.

CHAPTER 4: "JESUS NEVER SPOKE ABOUT HOMOSEXUALITY"

1. To be sure, I'm not suggesting that the preacher in Ecclesiastes was wrong when he stated that there was "nothing new under the sun." Instead, I'm suggesting that pastoral ministry requires us to read and apply the Bible in new situations as the needs of people arise. I believe this is what we see in the New Testament epistles on a regular basis.

2. For a great study on Jesus' relationship to Scripture, see John William Wenham, *Christ and the Bible* (Eugene, OR: Wipf & Stock, 2009).

3. I am well aware of the text-critical debate over the inclusion of John 8:2–11 in the gospel of John. From a text-critical standpoint, I would agree that this passage likely did not originally appear in John's gospel. I do, however, find Edward Klink's comments on the pericope to be helpful. While his commentary on the gospel of John offers a more expansive explanation regarding the difficulties surrounding the origins of this passage (and I would encourage you to read them), Klink gives a helpful conclusion as to how the passage can function for Christian's today. He writes, "Using an analogy, this pericope should be treated as a text on probation, given full membership without loss of rights or privileges, yet serving as if on an extended apprenticeship (which has lasted now for thirteen-hundred years). Just as a person on probation is prohibited from serving in certain authoritative capacities, so also might this text be prohibited from making its own contribution to a doctrine or theological issue. It can be used in collaboration with other pericopae in a secondary and supportive role but should not serve in an independent and isolated position of authority for the church. Such an approach allows it to function according to its verifiable nature without denying material concerns. While it is recommended that the pastor or teacher declare the (material) probationary status of this pericope to the church, to take away its full (functional) rights and privileges, in our opinion, only does more harm than good and only causes more confusion than certainty." Edward W. Klink III, *John*, Zondervan Exegetical Commentary on the New Testament, ed. Clinton E. Arnold (Grand Rapids, MI: Zondervan, 2016), 390.

4. Grant R. Osborne, *Matthew*, Zondervan Exegetical Commentary on the New Testament (Grand Rapids, MI: Zondervan, 2010), 197.

CHAPTER 5: CHRIST: "TO SEEK AND SAVE THE LOST"

1. Gordon J. Wenham, *Genesis 1–15*, vol. 1, Word Biblical Commentary (Dallas, TX: Word, Incorporated, 1987), 80.
2. Ibid., 81.
3. Victor P. Hamilton, *The Book of Genesis, Chapters 1–17*, The New International Commentary on the Old Testament (Grand Rapids, MI: Eerdmans, 1990), 207.
4. Many modern commentators are reluctant to tie this scene of the provision of animal skins to the forgiveness of sins that comes through atonement. This is typical of commentators and scholars who focus narrowly on the historical context of the passage without giving attention to the canonical and theological contexts in which the historical context is also embedded. I was once guilty of this narrow type of reading, but have learned that many, especially within the early and medieval church, saw no problem reading passages of Scripture in both a historical and theological context. I, for one, am now convinced that alongside our historical and grammatical interpretation of the Scriptures we should also pay attention to the canonical and theological contexts in which these Scriptures are received by the church. One example of the type of interpretation that I am advocating for here in this passage is seen in Martin Luther's comments about Genesis 3:21, where he wrote, "Thus they were to be constantly afraid of sinning, to repent continually, and to sigh for the forgiveness of sins through the promised Seed." *Luther's Works, Volume 1: Lectures on Genesis: Chapters 1–5* (St. Louis, MO: Concordia Publishing House, 1999), 221.
5. See chapters 3 and 4 in Tremper Longman, *Immanuel in Our Place: Seeing Christ in Israel's Worship*, The Gospel According to the Old Testament (Phillipsburg, NJ: P&R, 2001).
6. On this theme of God's relational presence, see J. Scott Duvall and J. Daniel Hays, *God's Relational Presence: The Cohesive Center of Biblical Theology* (Grand Rapids, MI: Baker Academic, 2019).
7. D. A. Carson, *Matthew 1–12*, The Expositor's Bible Commentary (Grand Rapids, MI: Zondervan Publishing, 1995), 25.
8. John R. W. Stott, *The Cross of Christ*, 20th anniversary ed. (Downers Grove, IL: IVP Books, 2006), 85.

CHAPTER 6: "GAY" CHRISTIANS—MORAL IDENTITY AND THE CHRISTIAN LIFE

1. Grant Macaskill, *Living in Union with Christ: Paul's Gospel and Christian Moral Identity* (Ada, MI: Baker Academic, 2023), viii.

2. Ibid.
3. Macaskill, viii–ix.
4. Macaskill, 40.
5. Macaskill, ix.
6. Thomas H. McCall, *Against God and Nature: The Doctrine of Sin*, Foundations of Evangelical Theology Series (Wheaton, IL: Crossway, 2019), 21.
7. Rachel Gilson, *Born Again This Way* (Epsom, UK: The Good Book Company, 2020), 135.
8. John Piper, "Foreword to 'Overcoming Sin and Temptation: Three Classic Works by John Owen,'" Desiring God, October 23, 2006, https://www.desiringgod.org/articles/foreword-to-overcoming-sin-and-temptation-three-classic-works-by-john-owen.

CHAPTER 7: "WILL WE SEE YOU AT THE WEDDING?"—GAY MARRIAGE

1. The five principles that follow are taken from my article, Casey B. Hough, "5 Ways to Love Your Gay Neighbor," The Ethics & Religious Liberty Commission, June 21, 2017, https://erlc.com/resource-library/articles/5-ways-to-love-your-gay-neighbor/.

CHAPTER 10: "MY DAUGHTER BELIEVES SHE'S MY SON"

1. "Gender Dysphoria Information | Mount Sinai—New York," Mount Sinai Health System, https://www.mountsinai.org/health-library/diseases-conditions/gender-dysphoria.
2. Debra Soh, *The End of Gender: Debunking the Myths About Sex and Identity in Our Society* (New York, NY: Threshold Editions, 2020), 141.
3. Cecilia Dhejne et al., "Long-Term Follow-Up of Transsexual Persons Undergoing Sex Reassignment Surgery: Cohort Study in Sweden," *PLOS ONE* 6, no. 2 (February 22, 2011): e16885, https://doi.org/10.1371/journal.pone.0016885.
4. Church history as well as our own observations remind us that we are still living on earth with its fallenness and all that entails—sin is very much present, though with the help of the Holy Spirit, believers will strive against it. Final victory over every sin may not come in our lifetime, but we have assurance that in heaven there will be no vestige of physical, mental, or emotional illness. Perhaps we can take comfort in knowing of the struggle of some of the greatest saints. For example, the great hymn writer William Cowper struggled with depression and anxiety. See John Piper, "Depression

Fought Hard to Have Him," *Desiring God*, November 26, 2019, https://www.desiringgod.org/articles/depression-fought-hard-to-have-him.

CHAPTER 12: YOU ARE HERE: OUR PLACE IN GOD'S REDEMPTIVE PLAN

1. David Briones, "Already, Not Yet: How to Live in the Last Days," August 4, 2020, Desiring God, https://www.desiringgod.org/articles/already-not-yet.

CHAPTER 13: BIRTHDAYS AND BATHROOMS— LIVING AS CHRISTIANS IN PUBLIC

1. Peter C. Craigie, *The Book of Deuteronomy*, The New International Commentary on the Old Testament (Grand Rapids, MI: Eerdmans, 1976), 169–70.

CONCLUSION: "AND SUCH WERE SOME OF YOU"

1. Anthony C. Thiselton, *The First Epistle to the Corinthians: A Commentary on the Greek Text*, New International Greek Testament Commentary (Grand Rapids, MI: Eerdmans, 2000).
2. Roy E. Ciampa and Brian S. Rosner, *The First Letter to the Corinthians*, The Pillar New Testament Commentary (Grand Rapids, MI: Eerdmans, 2010), 240.